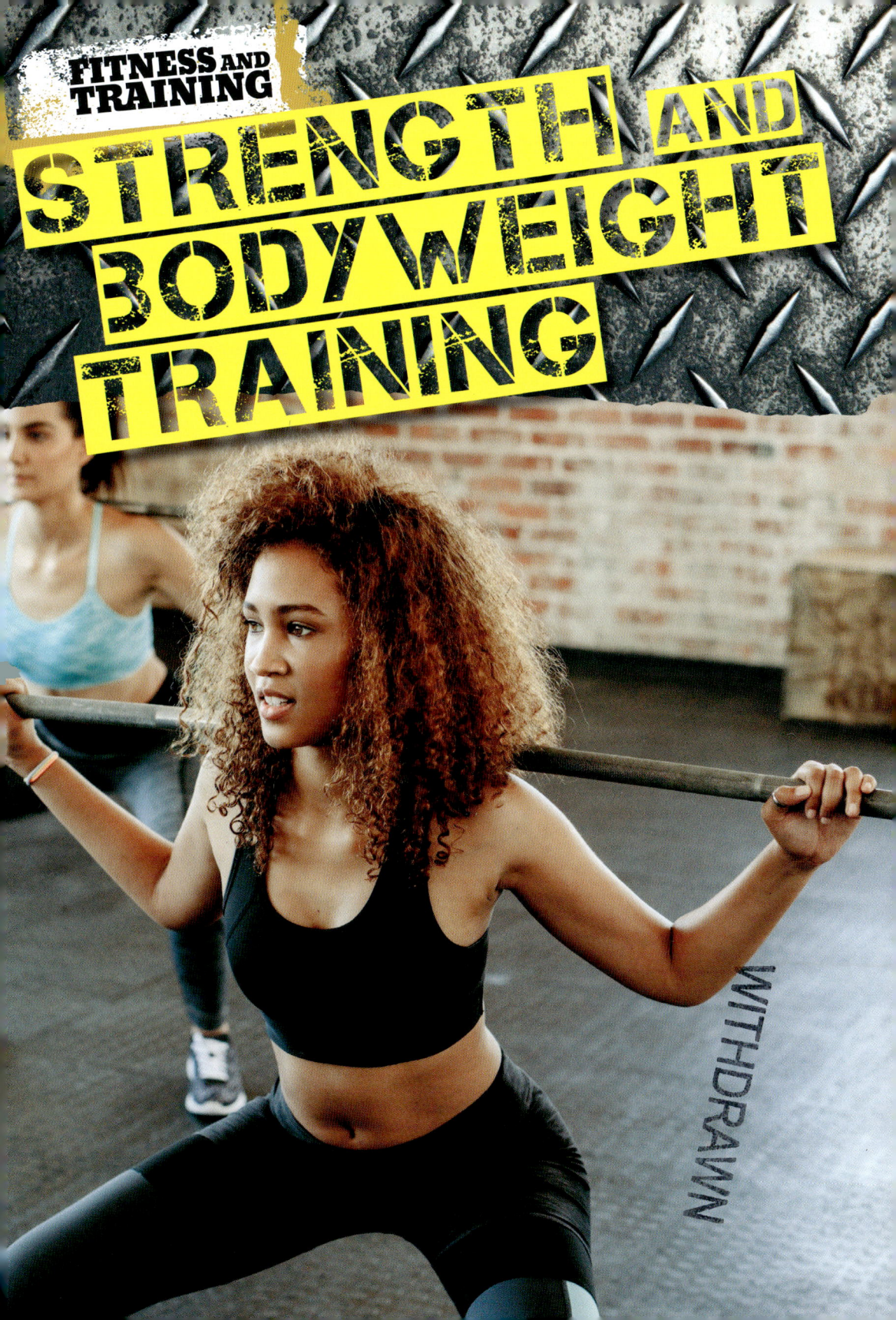

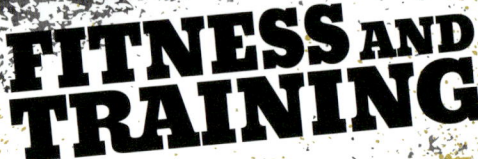

FITNESS AND TRAINING

Core Training
Endurance Training
Fitness and Nutrition
High-Energy Workouts
High-Intensity Interval Training (HIIT)
Low Impact Training
Mind and Body Fitness
Strength and Bodyweight Training

FITNESS AND TRAINING

STRENGTH AND BODYWEIGHT TRAINING

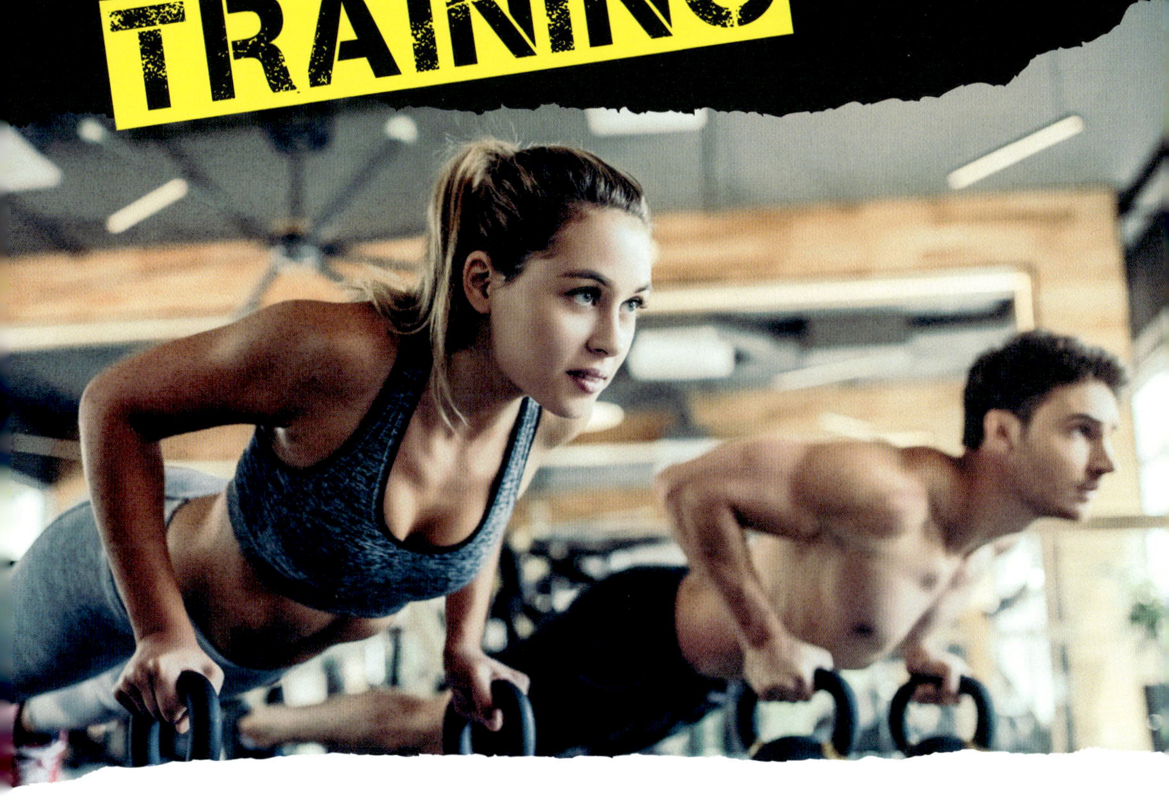

Kimber Rozier

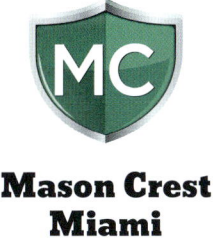

Mason Crest
Miami

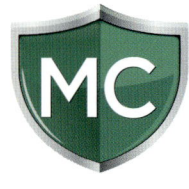

Mason Crest
PO Box 221876
Hollywood, FL 33022
(866) MCP-BOOK (toll-free)
www.masoncrest.com

Copyright © 2023 by Mason Crest, an imprint of National Highlights, Inc. All rights reserved. No part of this publication may be reproduced or transmitted in any form or by any means, electronic or mechanical, including photocopying, recording, taping, or any information storage and retrieval system, without permission from the publisher.

First printing
9 8 7 6 5 4 3 2 1
ISBN (hardback) 978-1-4222-4602-3
ISBN (series) 978-1-4222-4594-1
ISBN (ebook) 978-1-4222-7218-3

Library of Congress Cataloging-in-Publication Data

Names: Rozier, Kimber, author.
Title: Strength and bodyweight training / Kimber Rozier.
Description: Hollywood, FL : Mason Crest, 2023 |
 Series: Fitness and training | Includes bibliographical references and index.
Identifiers: LCCN 2020003315 | ISBN 9781422246023 (hardback) |
 ISBN 9781422272183 (ebook)
Subjects: LCSH: Weight training–Juvenile literature. |
 Isometric exercise–Juvenile literature. | Muscle strength–Juvenile literature.
Classification: LCC GV546.2 .R69 2021 | DDC 613.7/13–dc23
LC record available at https://lccn.loc.gov/2020003315

Developed and Produced by National Highlights, Inc.
Editor: Andrew Luke
Production: Crafted Content, LLC

QR CODES AND LINKS TO THIRD-PARTY CONTENT

You may gain access to certain third-party content ("Third-Party Sites") by scanning and using the QR Codes that appear in this publication (the "QR Codes"). We do not operate or control in any respect any information, products, or services on such Third-Party Sites linked to by us via the QR Codes included in this publication, and we assume no responsibility for any materials you may access using the QR Codes. Your use of the QR Codes may be subject to terms, limitations, or restrictions set forth in the applicable terms of use or otherwise established by the owners of the Third-Party Sites. Our linking to such Third-Party Sites via the QR Codes does not imply an endorsement or sponsorship of such Third-Party Sites or the information, products, or services offered on or through the Third-Party Sites, nor does it imply an endorsement or sponsorship of this publication by the owners of such Third-Party Sites.

CONTENTS

Chapter 1: The Importance of Strength Training 7
Chapter 2: Bodyweight Training 19
Chapter 3: The Science Behind Resistance Training 31
Chapter 4: Bodyweight Training vs. Weight Training 43
Chapter 5: Strength Training for Young Athletes 55
Chapter 6: Common Injuries and How to Prevent Them . . .67
Chapter 7: Strength Training Exercises 79
Series Glossary of Key Terms 92
Further Reading & Internet Resources 93
Index 94
Author Biography, Photo Credits & Educational Video Links . . 96

KEY ICONS TO LOOK FOR

WORDS TO UNDERSTAND: These words, with their easy-to-understand definitions, will increase readers' understanding of the text while building vocabulary skills.

SIDEBARS: This boxed material within the main text allows readers to build knowledge, gain insights, explore possibilities, and broaden their perspectives by weaving together additional information to provide realistic and holistic perspectives.

EDUCATIONAL VIDEOS: Readers can view videos by scanning our QR codes, providing them with additional educational content to supplement the text.

TEXT-DEPENDENT QUESTIONS: These questions send the reader back to the text for more careful attention to the evidence presented there.

RESEARCH PROJECTS: Readers are pointed toward areas of further inquiry connected to each chapter. Suggestions are provided for projects that encourage deeper research and analysis.

SERIES GLOSSARY OF KEY TERMS: This back-of-the-book glossary contains terminology used throughout this series. Words found here increase the reader's ability to read and comprehend higher-level books and articles in this field.

WORDS TO UNDERSTAND

dual-energy X-ray absorptiometry—a scanning apparatus using two X-ray beams to calculate fatty tissue, bone density, and muscle mass

endorphins—chemicals released by the central nervous system and pituitary gland that cause positive sensations

neuromuscular control—the ability to safely and accurately perform movements in specific patterns

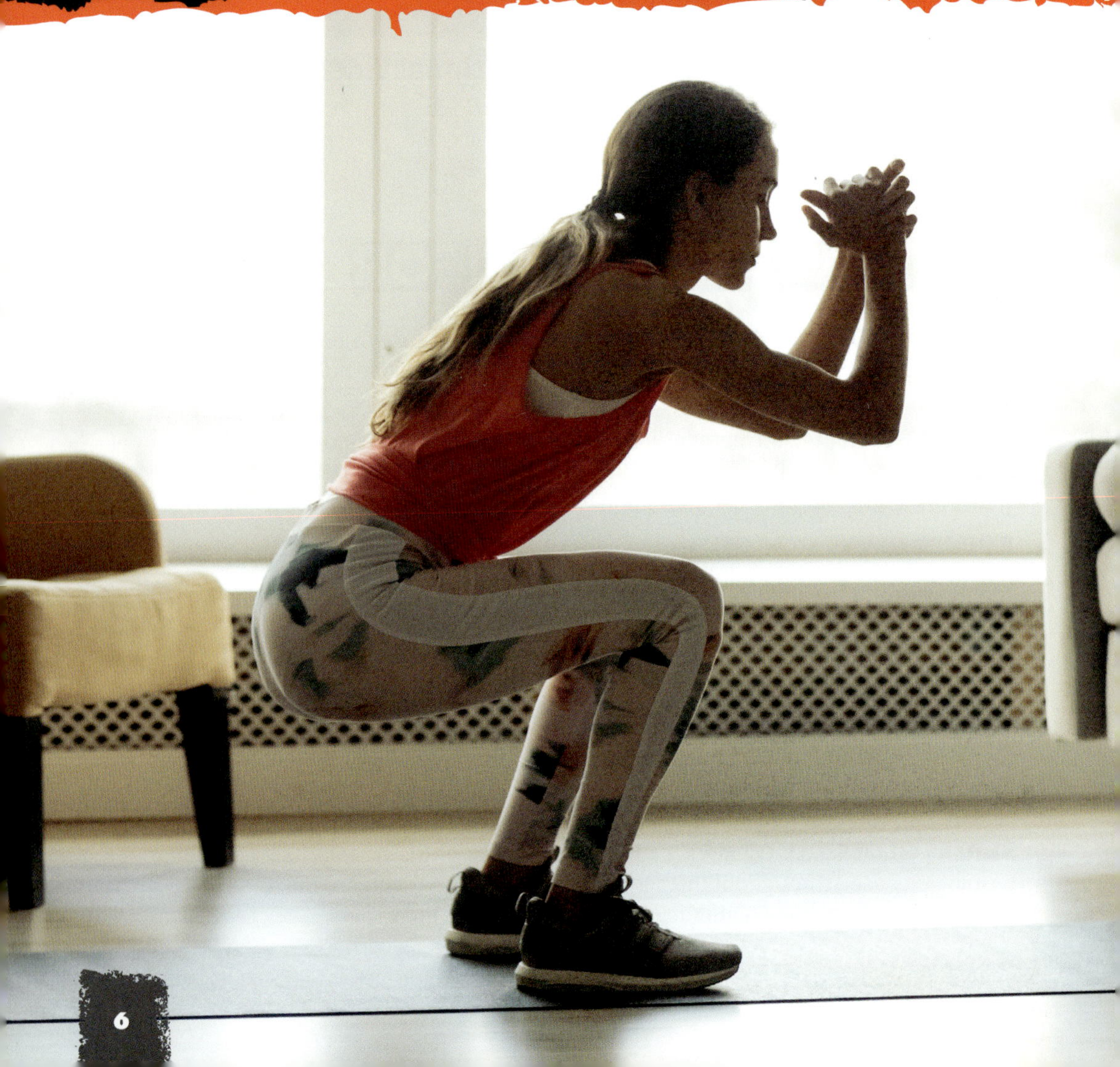

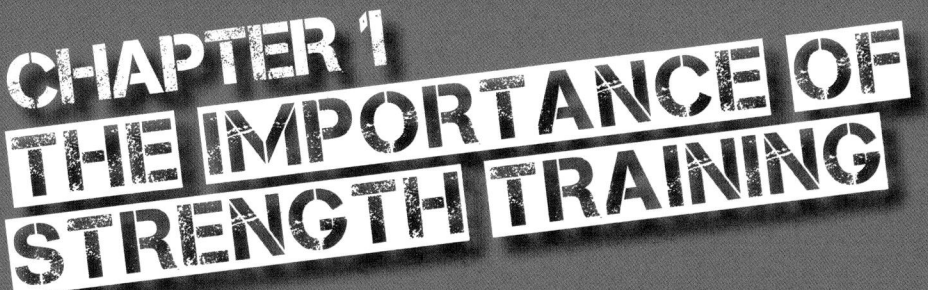

CHAPTER 1: THE IMPORTANCE OF STRENGTH TRAINING

When you think of strength training, what comes to mind? You're likely imagining a bodybuilder-type physique, lifting hundreds of pounds over his or her head. While this is only one sub-sector of the strength training community, we're often inundated with images of people doing heavy squats, barbell pressing, and guys pumped up on steroids.

Strength training is so much more than bodybuilding. In fact, it's important for everyone! Teenagers, in particular, have a lot to gain from weightlifting—and it isn't just muscle. A well-organized resistance training program provides a foundation for a healthy lifestyle into adulthood. It can also improve sports performance for youth athletes aiming to reach the next level.

The Benefits of Youth Strength Training

According to the National Strength and Conditioning Association, youth strength training provides the following health and wellness benefits:

- Reduced cardiovascular risk
- Improved bone health
- Motor-skill development
- Sports performance
- Injury prevention
- Better mood and psychological well-being

Therefore, you can use strength training regularly to take care of your all-around health.

Check out this video summarizing the benefits of strength training.

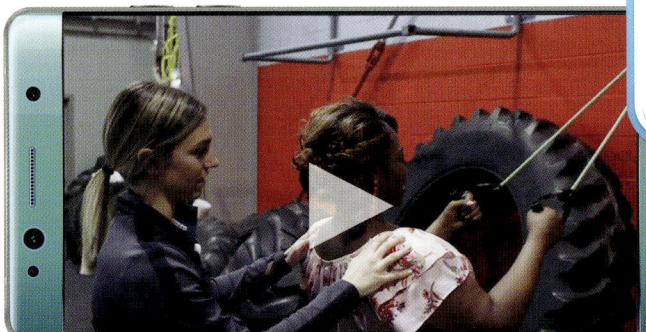

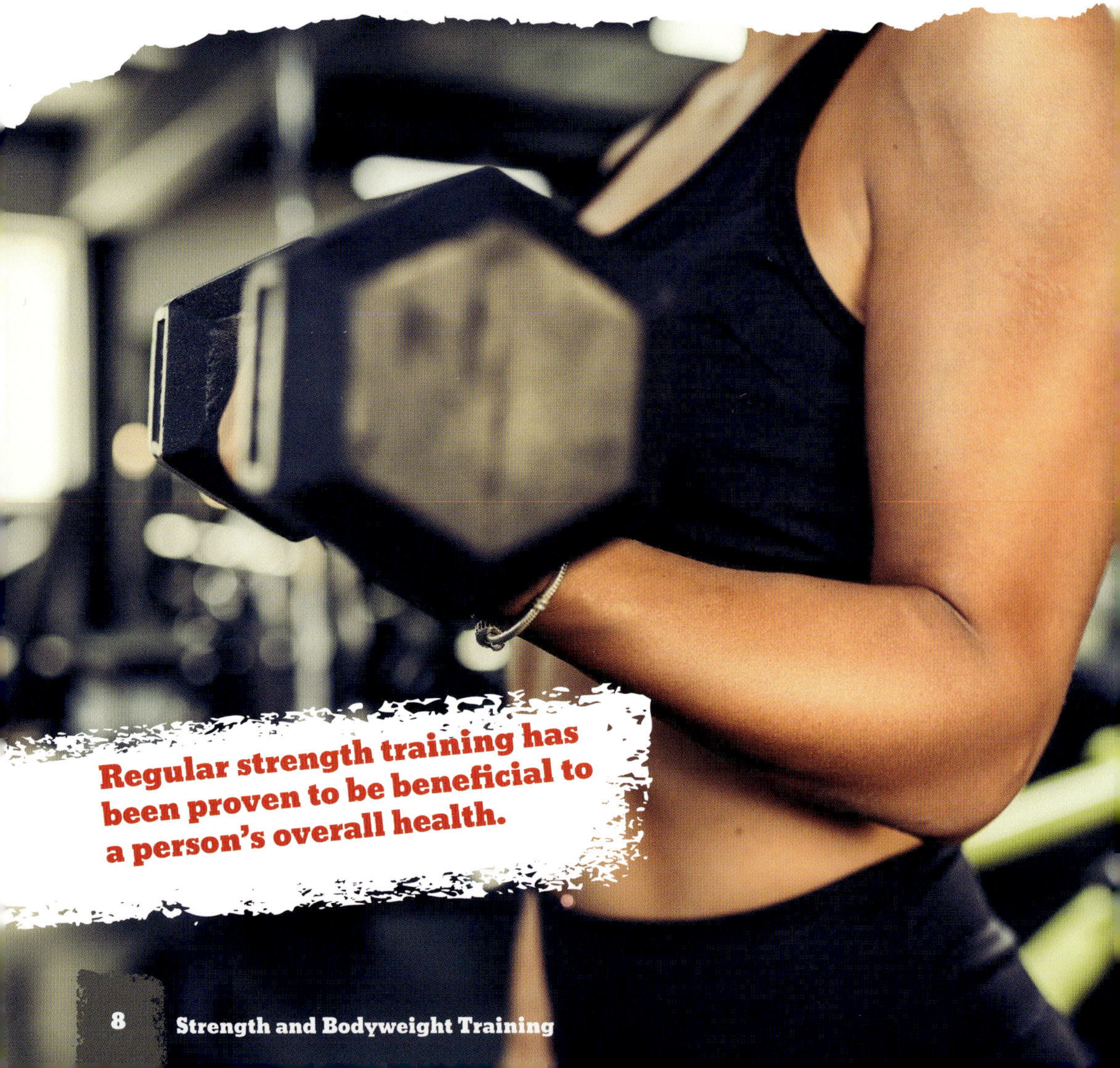

Regular strength training has been proven to be beneficial to a person's overall health.

The Effects of Strength Training on Body Composition

The overall amount of lean muscle mass, fat, water, and bone found in the human body is known as your body composition. Typically, it's measured as a ratio of fat mass to lean tissue, and it's often displayed simply as the percentage of body fat. Measuring body composition, therefore, is considered a marker of health in both adults and young people.

Without literally cutting into someone, however, it's impossible to measure body composition with complete accuracy. Instead, the current gold standard of measurement is **dual-energy X-ray absorptiometry**, or DEXA, the method that produces the most accurate measurements.

Lean Muscle Mass

Strength training shifts your body composition, helping it become more lean muscle mass dominant. Not only does weight training build muscle and burn fat during the workout, but it continues to work at rest. The more muscle you have, the better your metabolism functions to convert stored fat into energy. A healthy composition of lean body mass is associated with a reduced risk of diabetes, obesity, illness, and fracture.

Bone Density

Although once there was a concern about the effect strength training has on growth plates, that theory has since been debunked. In contrast, a supervised, well-organized, and appropriately progressive strength program can improve bone health across all ages. The mechanical stress placed upon bone during resistance training triggers processes that help bones form and grow stronger.

To optimize bone health, strength training should begin before puberty and continue into adulthood. According to research in the journal *Sports Medicine*, kids starting physical activity early experienced more stimulated bone and muscle growth compared with non-physically active youth.

CARDIO-VASCULAR HEALTH

If you consider cardio to only feature treadmills, ellipticals, and bike riding, you might be surprised to find that strength training helps your heart, too. Regular resistance training is correlated with a healthier heart in young people and it can play an important role in combating high cholesterol, inflammation, and insulin resistance.

As of 2019, the Centers for Disease Control cites cardiovascular disease as the leading cause of death in the United States. Accordingly, strength training offers a life-altering method to live longer and in better health. Moreover, the healthier your heart is, the easier it is to be active and get out there to enjoy life!

Neuromuscular Development

Neuromuscular control is a key developmental step. For example, crawling and ultimately learning to walk at a young age requires neuromuscular control to keep from falling over or getting injured. At its most basic, learning these skills requires a message from your brain to move, and it eventually receives feedback—either positive

The stress strength training puts on bones triggers processes that make them stronger.

or negative—about what happened. After a while, it makes small corrections to find the best, most efficient way to move. As such, these simple tasks eventually become routine and further development requires new challenges. Enter resistance training.

Young athletes tend to be deficient in jumping, landing, sprinting, and hand–eye coordination as they're still developing the proper neuromuscular function. Strength training provides a safe way to train and overload those patterns, reducing potential injury risk outside of the gym. Even non-sports-related movements, such as picking things up off the ground and reaching for items overhead, gain to benefit from strength training. Squats, push-ups, core exercises, and more train proper movement—especially when healthy patterns are taught from a young age.

STRENGTH TRAINING CAN SAVE LIVES

Did you know that 25–35% of American adults live a sedentary lifestyle? According to a longitudinal study conducted by the Aerobics Center, that factor alone has contributed to around 16% of all deaths since 1970. Researchers estimate that an inactive life doubles one's risk for developing a debilitating health condition. As physical activity becomes less of a functional necessity, it becomes even more important to get into the gym. Resistance training provides a fantastic way to counteract the rising issue of inactive lifestyles.

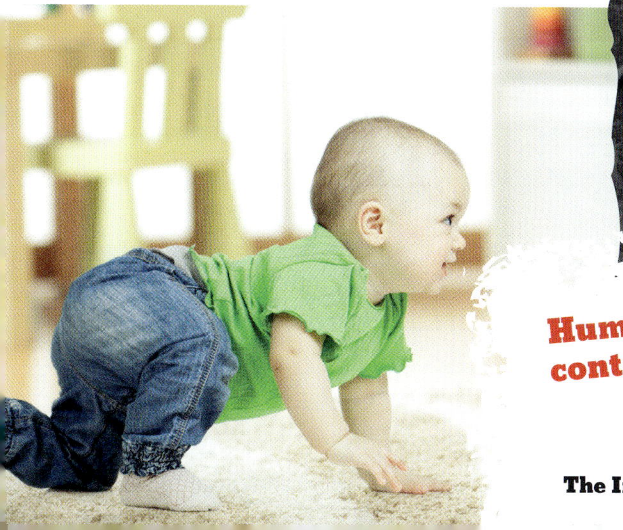

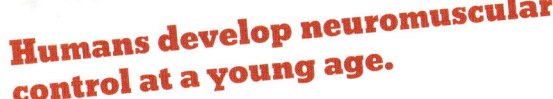

Humans develop neuromuscular control at a young age.

Growth and Maturation

As we've already mentioned, strength training provides crucial stimuli for maturation and growth in bones and muscles. A single session of strength training also stimulates two hormones involved in development—growth hormone and testosterone. Growth hormone, a chemical released by the pituitary gland in the brain, triggers bone and tissue growth as part of natural maturation. In boys, testosterone release corresponds with puberty, helping them mature into healthy young men. (Don't worry, girls—strength training won't turn you into a man. You don't have enough testosterone!)

Strength training is shown to stimulate growth hormone and testosterone.

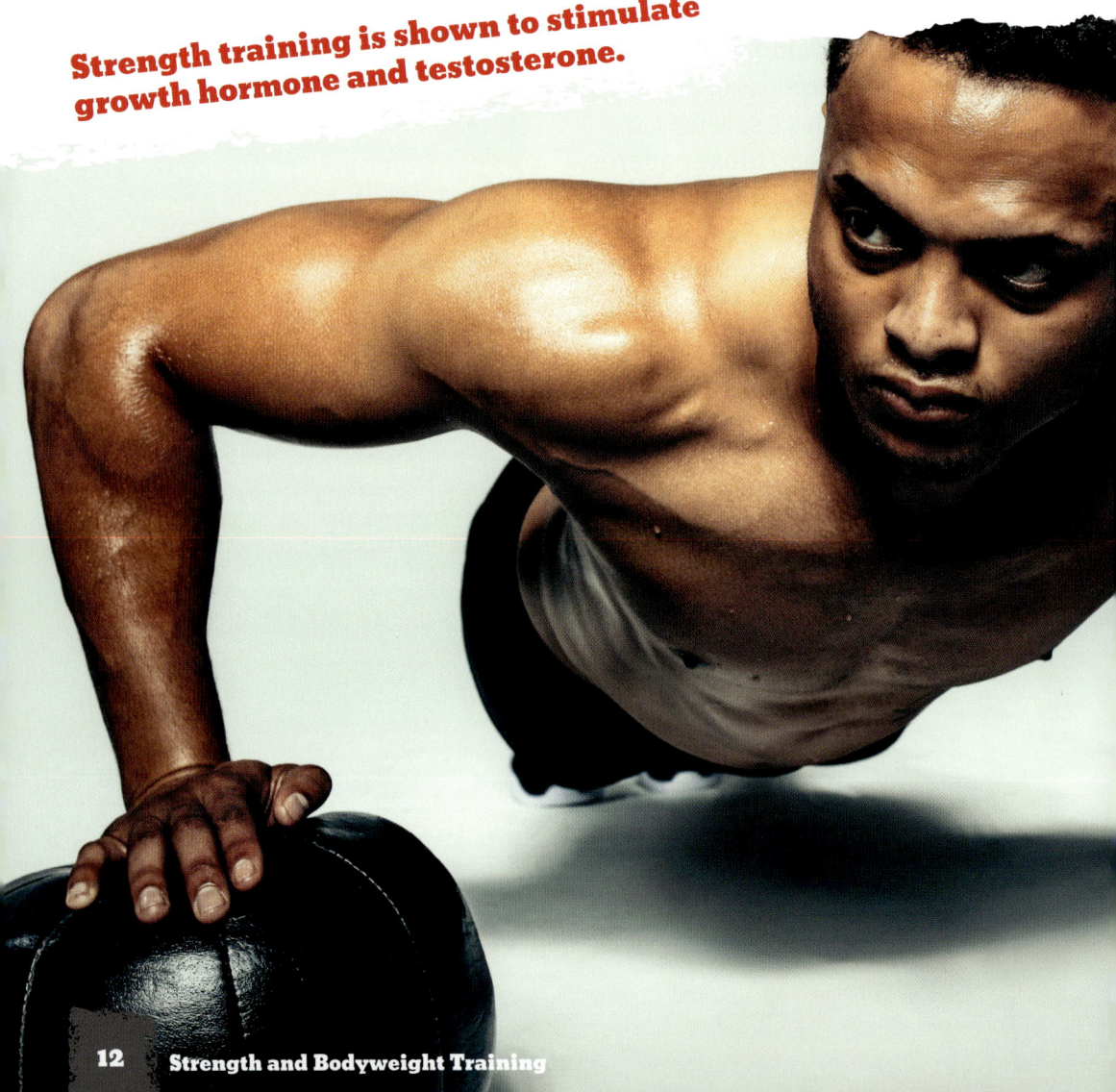

USE STRENGTH TRAINING TO OPTIMIZE MENTAL AND EMOTIONAL HEALTH

Exercise is known to release **endorphins**, but why is that important? The word endorphins forms a catchall term for any hormones in humans and other animals that produce a sensation of happiness. Interestingly, the word comes from a contraction of the words "endogenous" and "morphine," highlighting its ability to internally reduce the communication of pain and signal its opposite—euphoria. Endorphins are released from your central nervous system in response to laughter, food, physical intimacy, music, and of course, exercise. As completely natural and safe chemicals, the endorphins released by these activities provide a fantastic way to feel happy.

When it comes to exercise, however, endorphins are often associated with a "runner's high." But if you don't like running, are you doomed to never reap these rewards? On the contrary, in fact. Strength training offers an effective alternative for otherwise sedentary people who simply don't want to do aerobics. Arguably the most important aspect of strength training is to build healthy habits that carry into adulthood. Strength training a few times per week is one of the best ways to stay in shape. With mental and emotional health concerns becoming a national epidemic, the younger you start, the more prepared you'll be to combat them.

Cognitive Health

Another striking benefit of exercise that has emerged in recent years is its ability to make you smarter. Regular physical activity improves working memory as well as speeds up information processing. With rats as test subjects, one study published in the *Journal of Applied Physiology* even found that strength training alters the brain's cellular environment. By attaching little weights to the animals, researchers found that regular weighted ladder climbs reduced age-related memory loss. Therefore, resistance training could help you study for tests throughout high school, into college, and beyond.

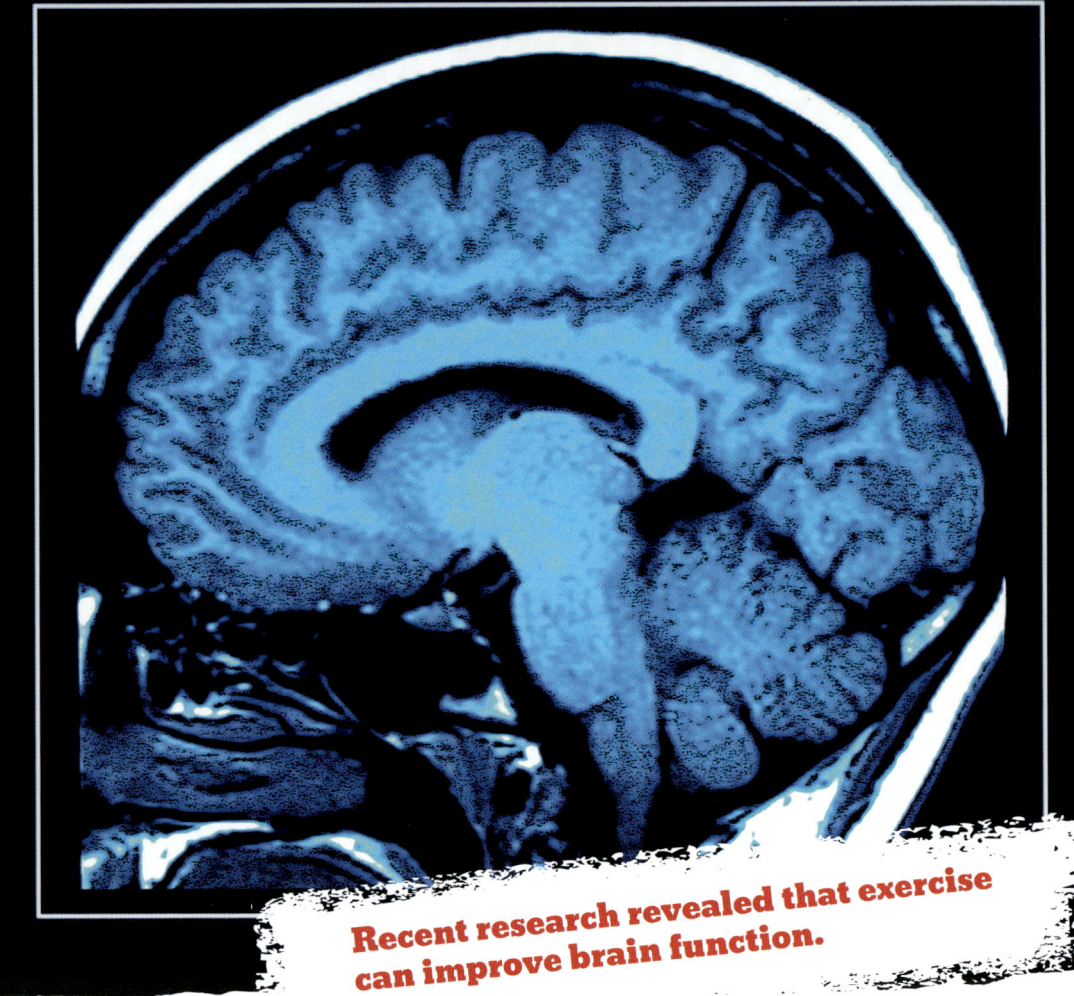

Recent research revealed that exercise can improve brain function.

Mental and Emotional Health

Well-being goes so far beyond basic physical condition. Mental and emotional health are just as important, and any issues should be treated with equal care. According to the World Health Organization, depression is one of the leading causes of illness across the globe. Furthermore, one in six people between ages 10 and 19 suffer from some type of mental or emotional illness. Just like you brush your teeth, eat good food, sleep, and exercise to avoid physical illness, the same amount of hygiene applies to psychological wellness.

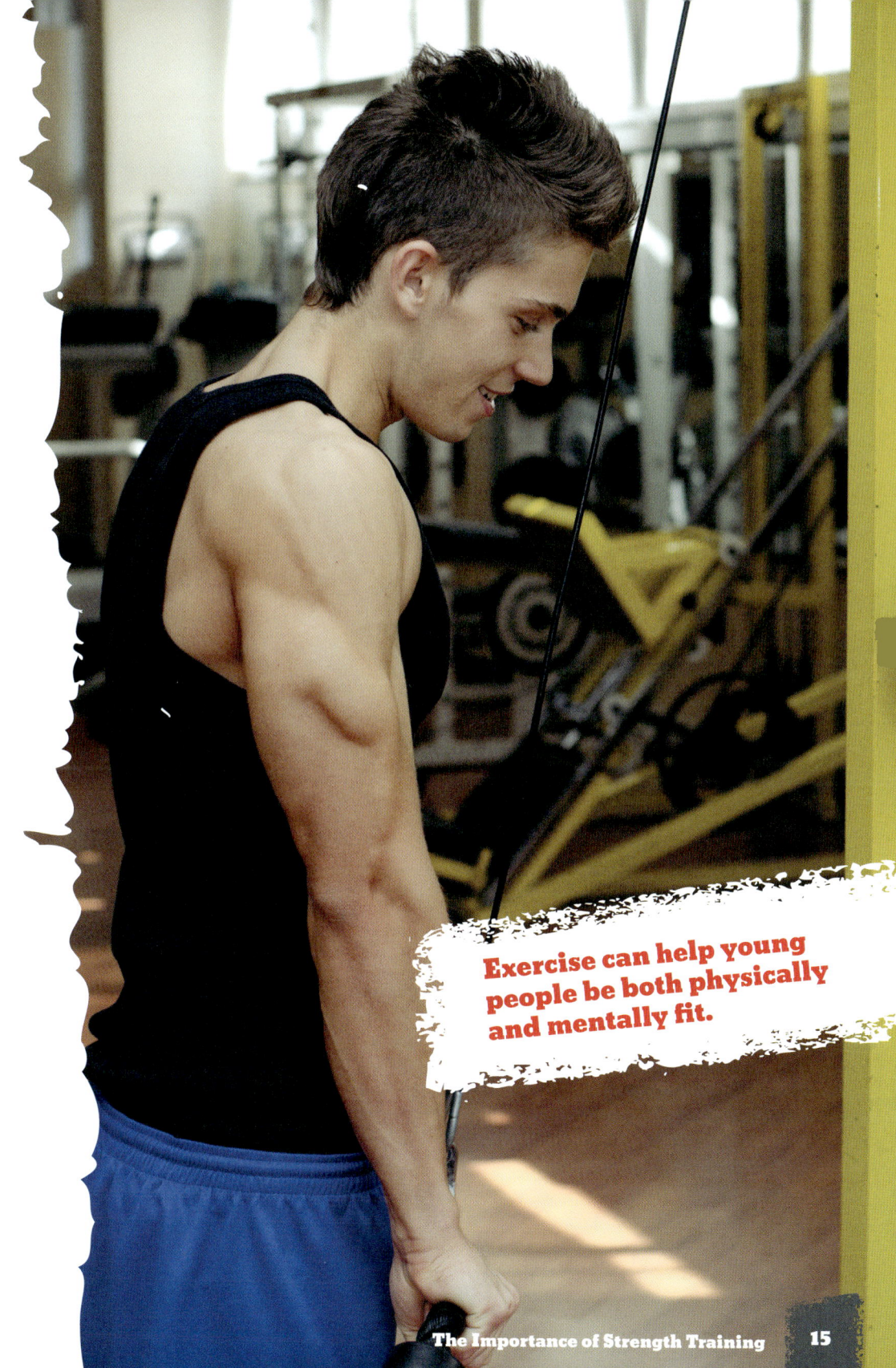

Exercise can help young people be both physically and mentally fit.

Learning to control your own body weight first is good training for moving on to other strength exercises.

In multiple cases, strength training has been linked to improved symptoms of depression, elevating mood and fostering interest in other activities. One study even showed benefits regardless of weekly frequency or amount of strength gained. It seems that simply getting out and doing the activity itself improved symptoms. Additionally, strength training has been shown to fight anxiety. When researchers at the University of Georgia looked at its effects versus either aerobic exercise or a control group, strength training calmed feelings of worry most effectively. While strength training is not a "cure" in the traditional sense, it can play a critical role in improving quality of life.

To repeat an important note—none of these benefits indicate that strength training cures mental illness. If you or anyone you know is struggling, check out the Internet Resources section at the end of this book for further assistance.

When beginning a strength training program, start with bodyweight training first. You need to be able to control yourself well before trying to control something else. Plus, bodyweight movements are always functional. Squatting down to pick something up, reaching overhead, and stepping over obstacles happens every day.

TEXT-DEPENDENT QUESTIONS

1. What are five benefits of resistance training?
2. What is neuromuscular control?
3. How does resistance training affect our mental health? Name three specific ways.

RESEARCH PROJECT

Resistance training is clearly important for all areas of health and wellness, but it's not the only form of exercise. Put together a chart comparing and contrasting the health benefits of resistance training, running, playing sports, and other forms of exercise.

WORDS TO UNDERSTAND

closed kinetic chain—describes exercises that lock your arms or legs in place while your body moves freely
open kinetic chain—describes exercises that allow free movement of the limbs
plyometrics—exercises involving quick muscular contractions designed to improve power, such as jumping or hopping
proprioception—the awareness of our body's position and movement in space

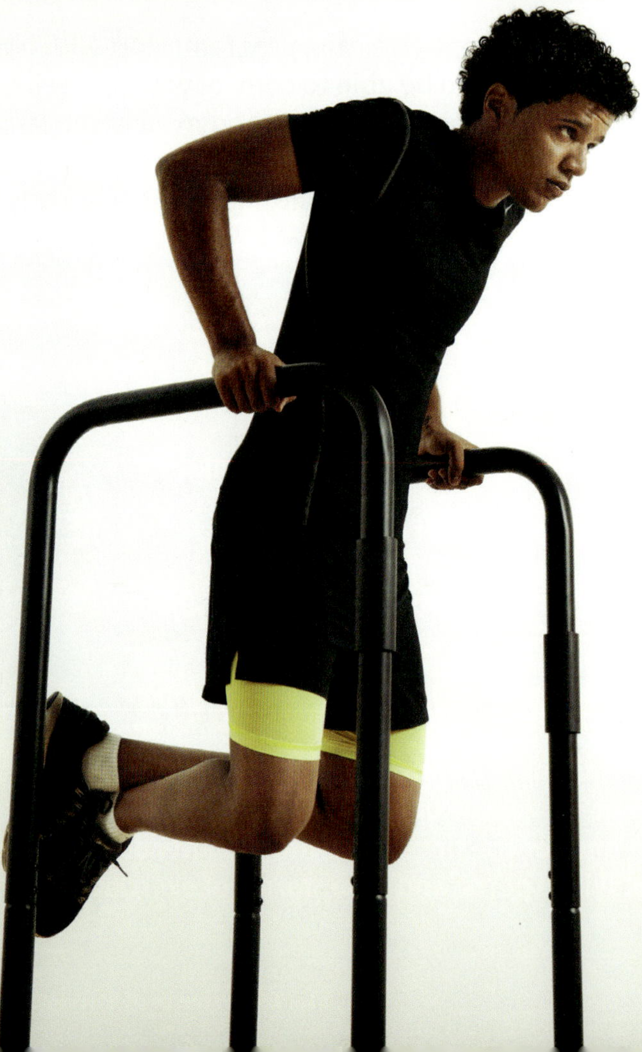

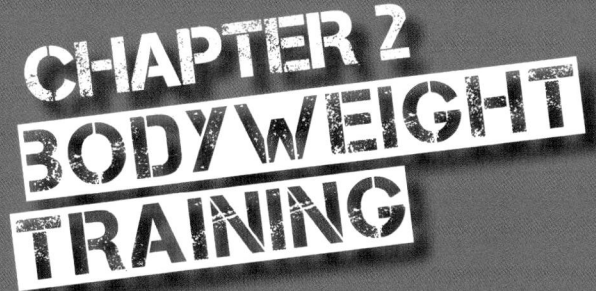

Chapter 2: Bodyweight Training

Bodyweight training involves a series of strength exercises using your own body to move against the natural resistance of gravity. You might not always be aware of it, but gravity is constantly pushing you down. By doing a bodyweight exercise, you're challenging your muscles to overcome that force to move your body.

Who Is It For?

Bodyweight training can help all ages and experience levels build core strength, stability, and total body muscle. While the breadth of bodyweight exercises can certainly produce results, they're not always ideal for every population. For example, pregnant women are advised to stay away from burpees due to impact on the stomach. Additionally, some overweight adults might find it difficult to control their entire body weight. Fortunately, adaptations are available for most situations.

The Benefits of Bodyweight Training

Obviously, the amount of weight you have to move depends on your size. However, we can manipulate gravity to make bodyweight exercises harder or easier. Therefore, one of the primary benefits of bodyweight training is the ease of execution.

Other benefits of bodyweight training include:

> Increased strength
> Improved **proprioception**
> Better coordination
> Conditioning applications

Regardless of your experience, you can use your body weight to get stronger. The harder you ask your muscles to work, the stronger you'll get. For example, the military uses push-ups, pull-ups, and crunches—all bodyweight movements—to test strength.

BODYWEIGHT TRAINING ADDS FUNCTIONAL MUSCLE

You know what they say—you can't build a house without a strong foundation. Cutting the basics short in favor of more "impressive"

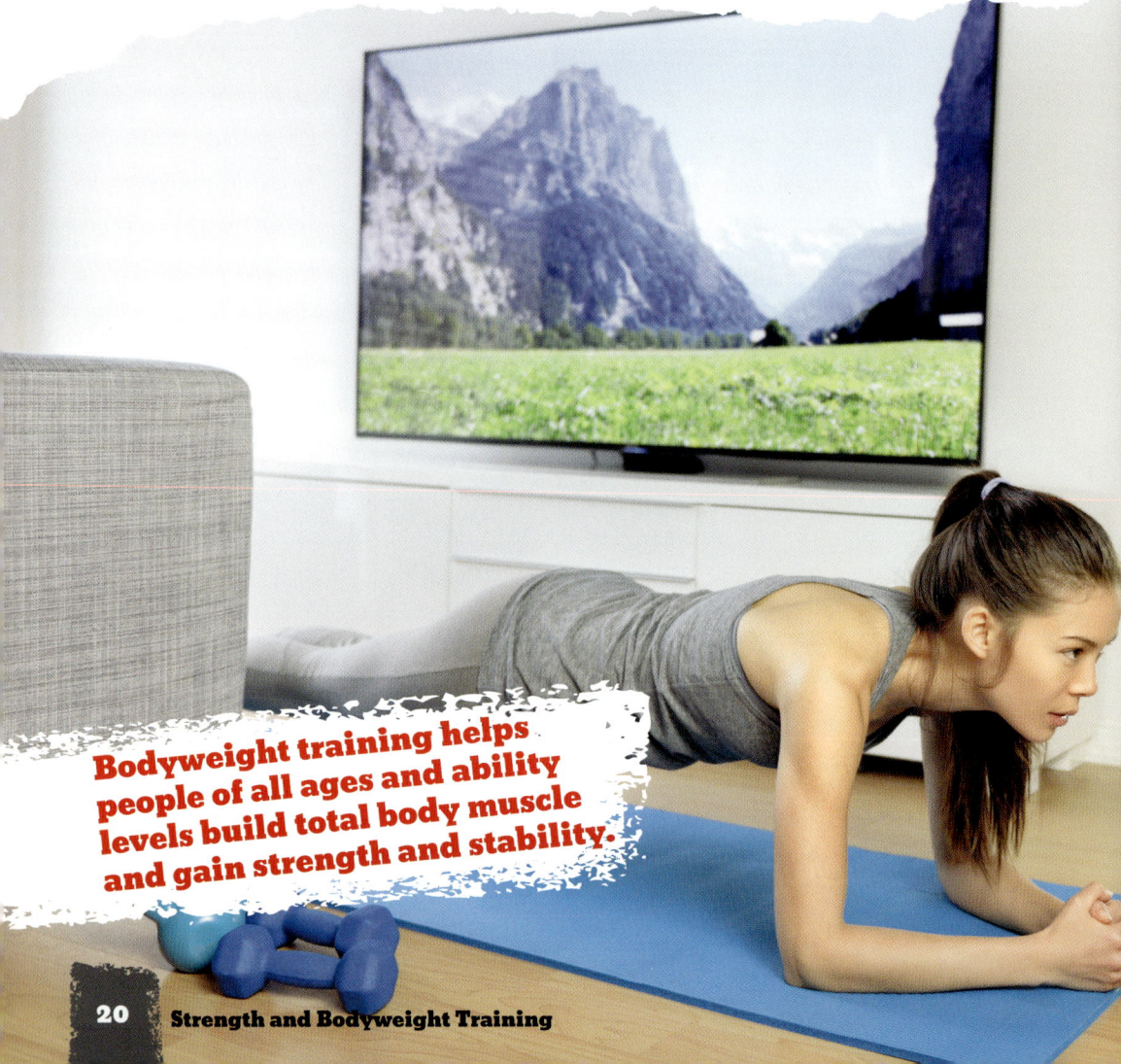

Bodyweight training helps people of all ages and ability levels build total body muscle and gain strength and stability.

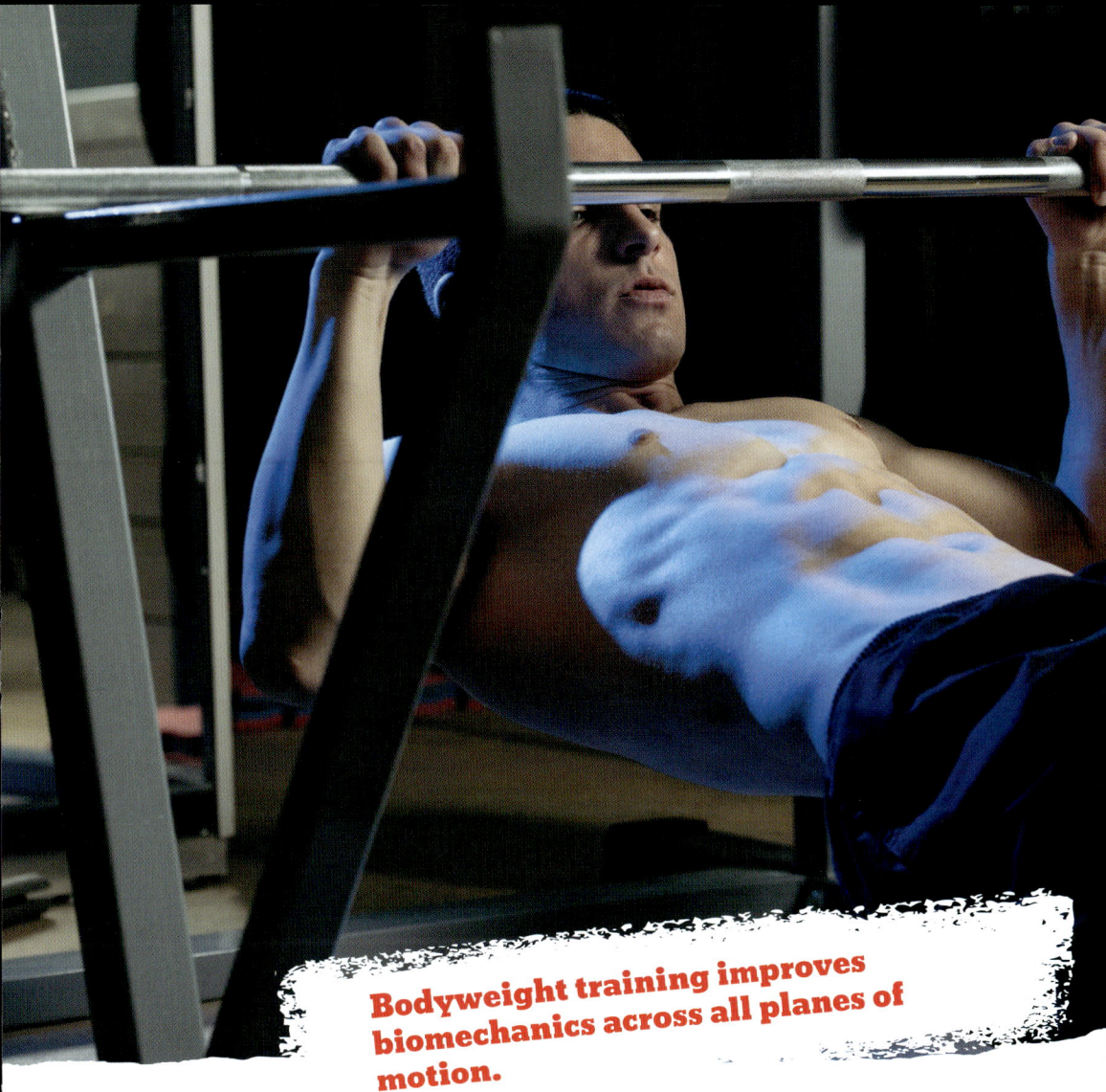

Bodyweight training improves biomechanics across all planes of motion.

exercises will only reduce results in the long-term. It's like trying to skip to graduate-level courses before learning basic math. Ultimately, it's a waste of time.

Oddly enough, being able to control your body across multiple planes is a skill everyone is born with. Unfortunately, sitting at school all day, causes the loss of some of those natural abilities. Bodyweight training can help you practice sound biomechanics across all planes of motion, so you can regain a strong foundation and go even further.

Closed vs. Open Kinetic Chain Movements

A large majority of bodyweight exercises are **closed kinetic chain** movements. These are exercises that lock your arms or legs in place while your body moves freely. For example, in a squat, your feet are glued to the ground while your body descends and ascends. Closed kinetic chain bodyweight exercises require more coordination, as they necessitate controlled neuromuscular patterns. Basically, there's less room for error—if you can't control yourself, you either won't move, you'll fall over, or you'll open the chain somehow. As such, these types of exercises stimulate proprioception—the awareness of our body's position and movement in space.

Examples of closed-chain bodyweight exercises include:

> Push-ups
> Pull-ups
> Squats
> Split squats
> Inverted rows
> Romanian deadlifts
> Glute bridges

Open kinetic chain exercises, on the other hand, allow for free mobility of your limbs. Typically, these include movements designed to increase range of motion at a joint or improve strength in one specific muscle. While you can perform bodyweight exercises with an open kinetic chain, they're best used to aid mobility in a warm-up or cooldown. Why? Well, we're already really strong at moving our limbs without any extra resistance. It's what you did to brush your teeth, pick up your bag, and step out of the door today.

Does that make training them useless? Of course not! Boxing, for example, is a fantastic way to train the arms without any weights. Running involves open kinetic chain movement of the legs, and that can definitely get tiring. They're also great for rehabilitation. However, in the absence of injury, illness, or other abnormality, most open-chain bodyweight movements won't make you much stronger. Therefore, we don't typically associate them with strength training.

Examples of open-chain bodyweight exercises:

> Reverse fly
> Arm circles
> Bicycle crunches
> Side-lying leg raises
> Donkey kicks
> Flutter kicks

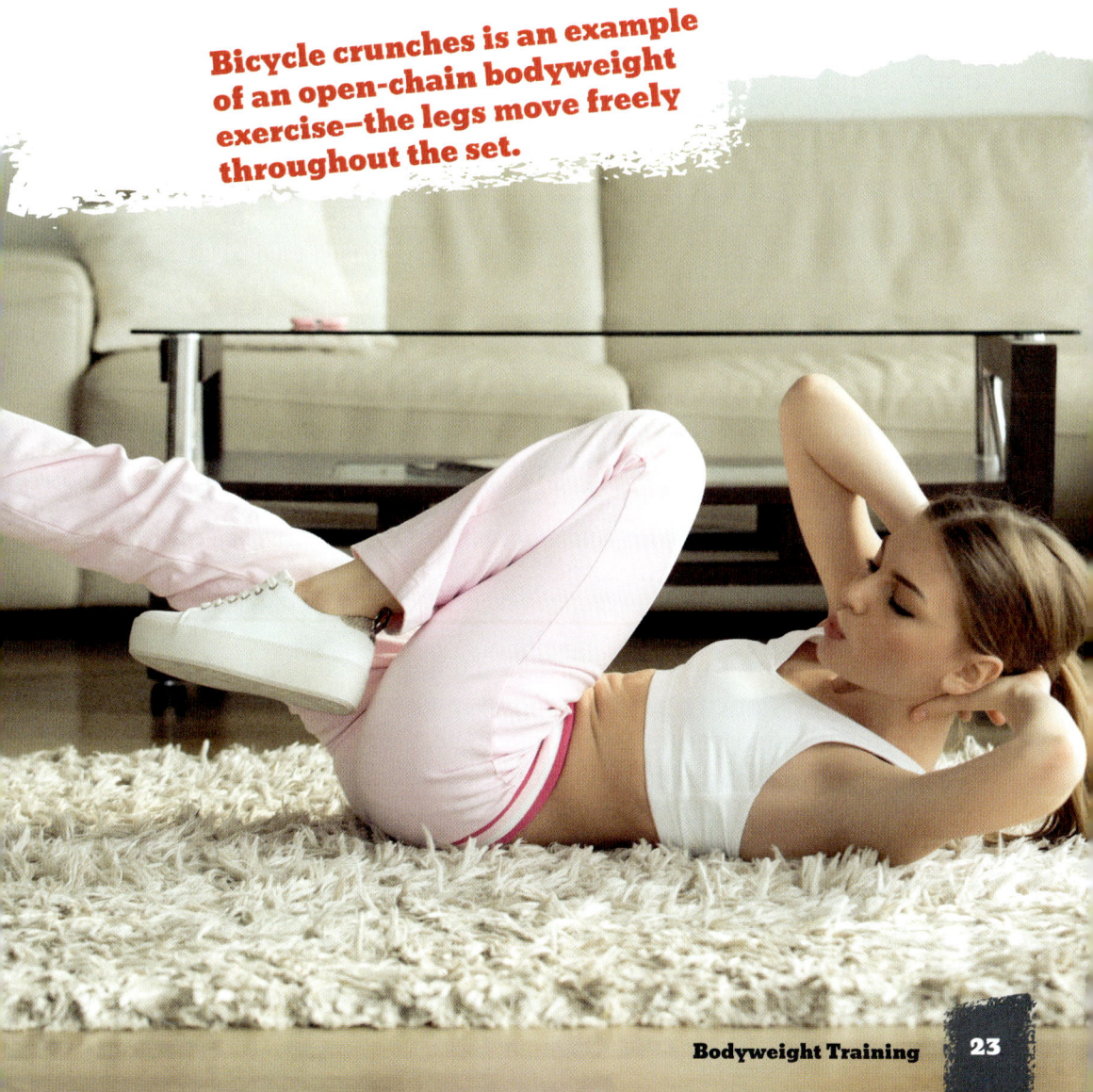

Bicycle crunches is an example of an open-chain bodyweight exercise—the legs move freely throughout the set.

Building Total Body Strength with Bodyweight Exercises

A full-extension, top-to-bottom pull-up is one of the best ways to test relative strength or how strong you are for your body weight. Once you've achieved one, you can continue to use them to increase upper body strength. Manipulating repetitions (reps), tempo, and grip targets different areas of back and arm musculature, and the same factors apply to other areas of the body.

For lower body strength, a full bodyweight squat is a perfect way to start. It demonstrates control, mobility, stability, and enough relative strength to overcome gravity. Yet, given that we spend most of our lives supporting our weight with our legs, bodyweight squats become easy quickly.

CONQUERING THE PULL-UP: THE EASIEST, MOST DIFFICULT EXERCISE

A pull-up is one of the simplest bodyweight exercises, yet it's incredibly hard to do! Why? Because a pull-up moves straight up and down, you're directly fighting gravity to pull your entire body upward. By slightly changing the angle, you can make it easier. Try lowering the bar to belly-button height. Then, you can grab on tight and lean back (while keeping your feet on the ground) for a much easier pulling exercise!

An easy way to progress is moving to one leg. It will immediately double the resistance placed upon the muscles of that leg. Obviously, it's also harder to balance. Therefore, start by supporting the second leg. Split squats and lunges work wonders, and you can even elevate the back leg to increase the demands of gravity. Continue to adjust the speed, add more reps, or manipulate the angle to get stronger.

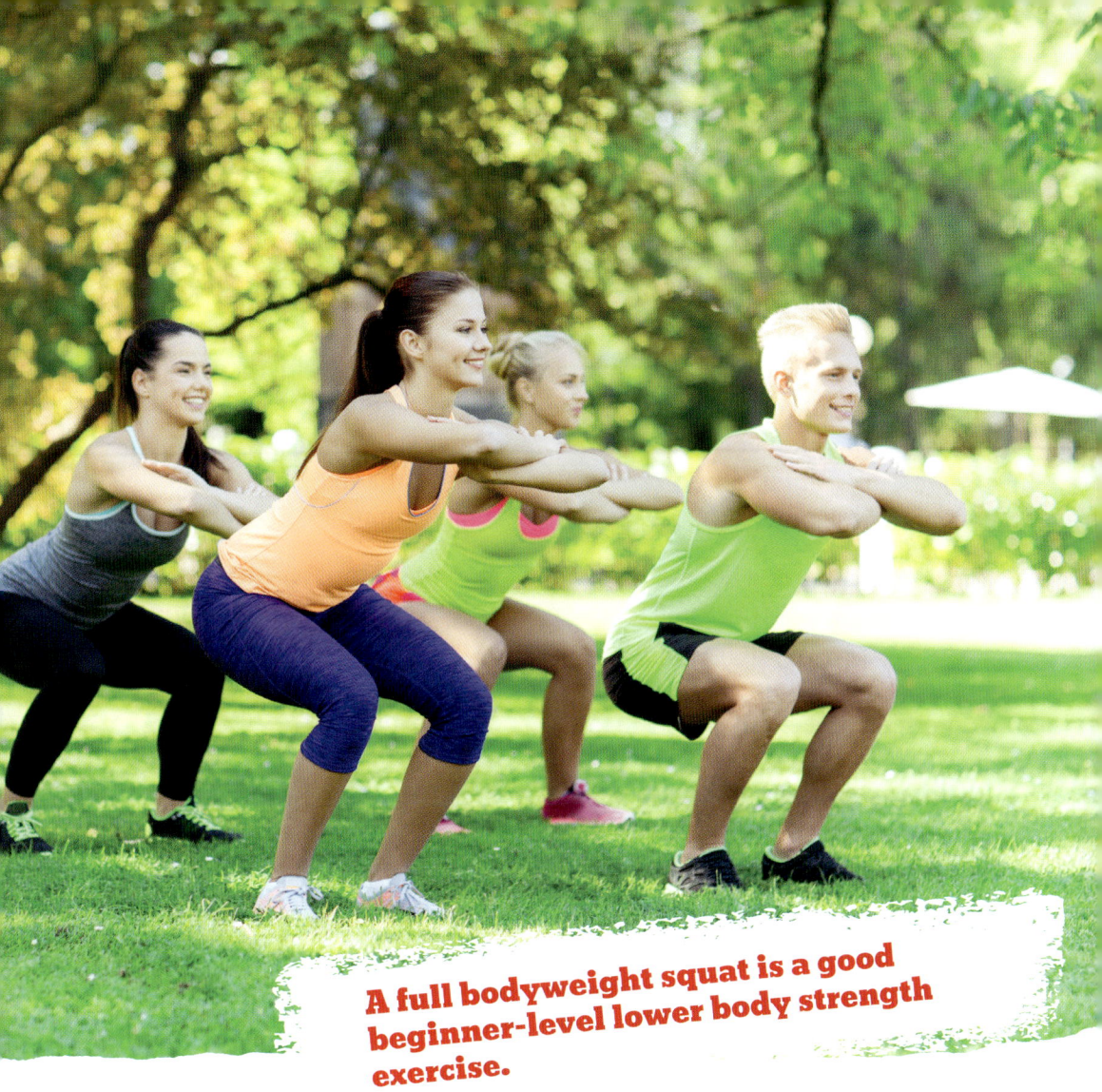

A full bodyweight squat is a good beginner-level lower body strength exercise.

USING YOUR OWN BODY WEIGHT TO DEVELOP POWER

Defined as exercises involving quick muscular contractions designed to improve power, such as jumping or hopping, **plyometrics** are a great way for an athlete to develop power and athleticism.

Jumping, landing, and cutting are integral to youth sports. Therefore, these movements should be trained for. Think of plyometrics as the most advanced version of bodyweight resistance training. It takes a great deal of coordination, balance, and strength to execute these movements at high speed. Just like you learn how to crawl before you walk, you can also learn how to and safely before you jump.

For example, when dropping down from a small height, aim for a stable, soft landing over the middle of both feet, similar to a squat position. Once you've mastered that, land on one leg. There are infinite progressions, but it's important to stick to the fundamentals first. Proper technique will prevent injury, especially at high impact.

Once you've learned how to land, move on to box jumps, vertical jumps, and broad jumps. These will teach your body to both be explosive and to absorb force without needing a gym. As you've probably been jumping around for years, these are skills that you already have. Therefore, something that takes very little time to refine yields huge results.

STRENGTHENING THE CORE—ONE OF THE MOST UNDERRATED BENEFITS OF BODYWEIGHT TRAINING

Push-ups, crawling, and single-leg movements all require stability. Guess where that stability comes from? Your core, of course.

Since it's just you and your body, bodyweight training provides ample opportunity to receive feedback about your posture. One thing you'll hear a lot throughout this book are the concepts of "bracing your core" and "maintaining a neutral spine." These phrases involve activating the muscles between your hips and your shoulders to stabilize movement.

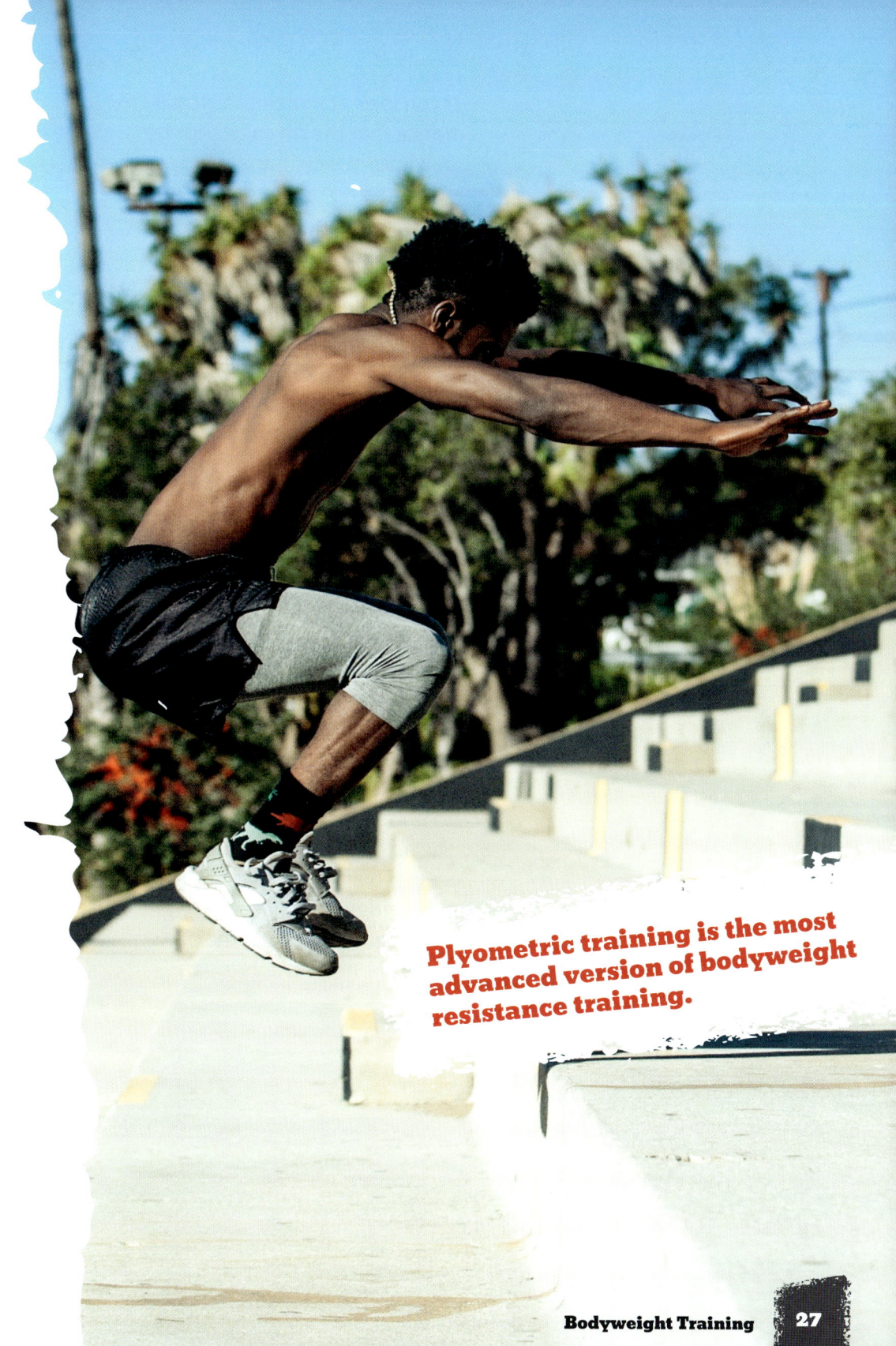

Plyometric training is the most advanced version of bodyweight resistance training.

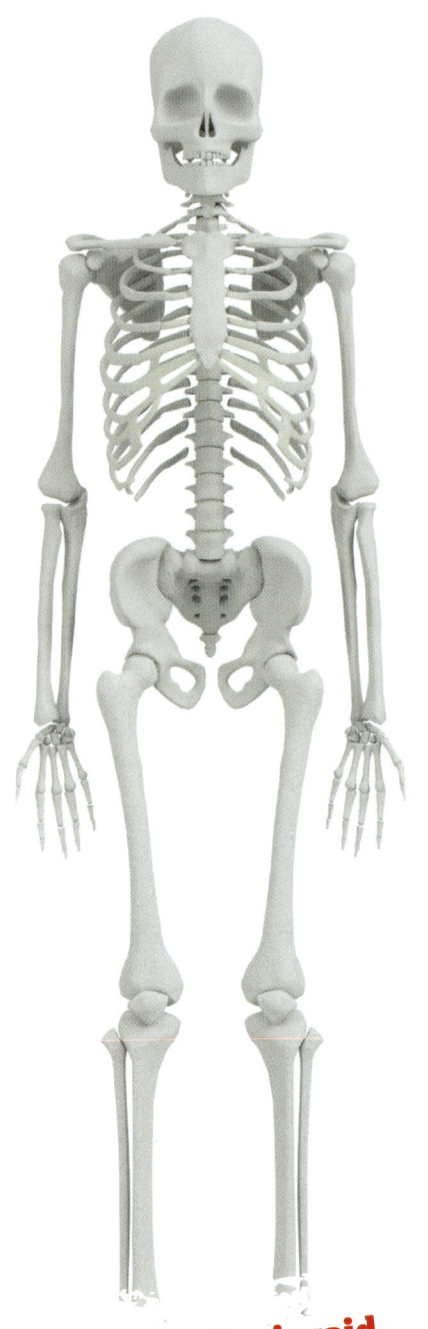

If you look at a skeleton, you'll notice that the rib cage and the pelvis form a cylindrical shape when stacked atop one another. Due to our natural anatomy, this is what it looks like when our spine is in neutral. Sometimes, when we move, these two ends move in different directions. The ribs flare out, our pelvis tilts, and our spine has to curve more than it's used to. This puts our spine in a compromised position, as it decreases the space to absorb force. However, when we brace our core, those muscles turn on and pull everything back into place. From a neutral position, our arms and legs can move freely while minimizing spinal injury risk.

In order to do a proper push-up, your legs and arms are locked into the ground. Therefore, you have to brace your core. If you don't, it's really easy to notice—your glutes will shoot into the air or your back will arch. The same goes for planks, side planks, and bridges. Using bodyweight training, therefore, is the perfect way to train a neutral spine.

A neutral spine is said to be achieved when the rib cage and the pelvis align like a cylinder.

Learn what a neutral spine is and why finding it is important in this video.

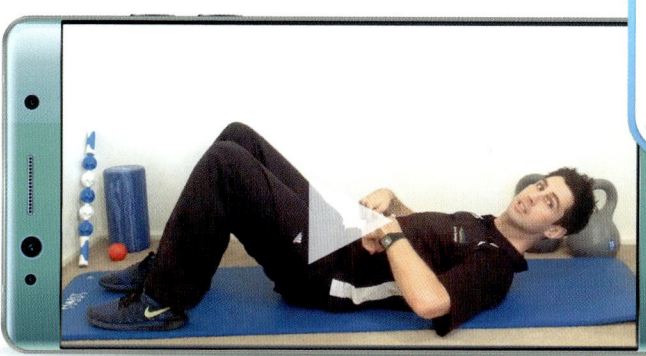

TEXT-DEPENDENT QUESTIONS

1. What are the benefits of closed-chain exercises?

2. What is a neutral spine, and why is it important?

3. How can you make a bodyweight exercise more difficult?

RESEARCH PROJECT

Many people believe you can't put on muscle mass without weights. Research bodyweight bodybuilding, and write a 500-word essay on what it is, how it works, and techniques to build muscle using only your body.

WORDS TO UNDERSTAND

actin and myosin—two proteins found in muscle tissue that help contraction

force-velocity curve—a graphical curve that represents the inverse relationship between force and velocity, often used as a basis to program intensities in resistance training

hypertrophy—the enlargement of the physical size of muscle tissue

SAID principle—a physiological principle stating that the human body adapts to the specific demands placed upon it

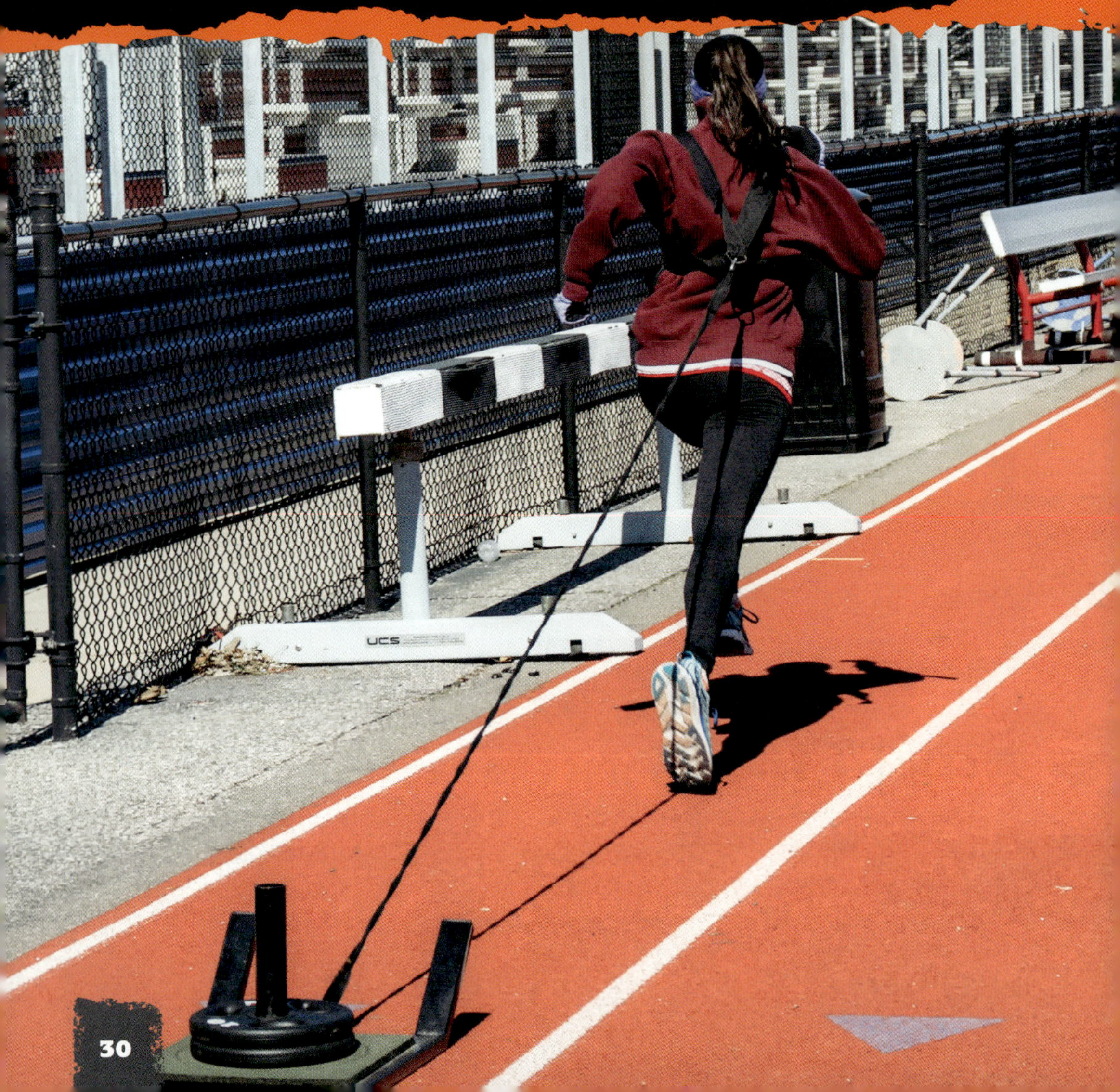

CHAPTER 3
THE SCIENCE BEHIND RESISTANCE TRAINING

We all know resistance training can make you bigger, faster, and stronger. The question is how does it work? In this chapter, we'll get into the science behind resistance training, so that you're armed with the understanding you need to apply these principles in real-life.

IT ALL STARTS FROM THE TOP—MOTOR UNIT RECRUITMENT

Before your muscles can contract, your brain has to tell them to do so. Therefore, there exists a strong connection between motor neurons and the muscle fibers they innervate. Muscle fibers are grouped in little teams called motor units, and each unit has a motor neuron that they report to. Some units are smaller, some are bigger, but once their motor neuron says it's time to work, all fibers within that unit contract.

Your body is smart and efficient, so it doesn't like to recruit more motor units than it needs. For smaller tasks, it uses its smaller units. Therefore, you might get a weaker yet effective contraction. During strength training, however, loads vary. With larger loads, you need more and larger motor units. That's why heavier lifting demands more work.

MUSCLE CONTRACTION

Muscle contraction involves tiny proteins called **actin and myosin.** Similar to oars on a rowboat, these filaments attach to each other and pull your muscles along. With each stroke, you get further and further. Each contraction requires energy and force production, which is what ultimately leaves you tired after a workout.

 This short video explains how muscle contraction works.

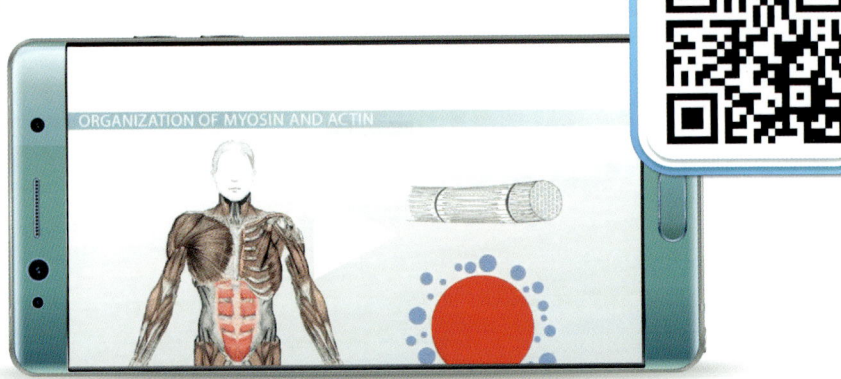

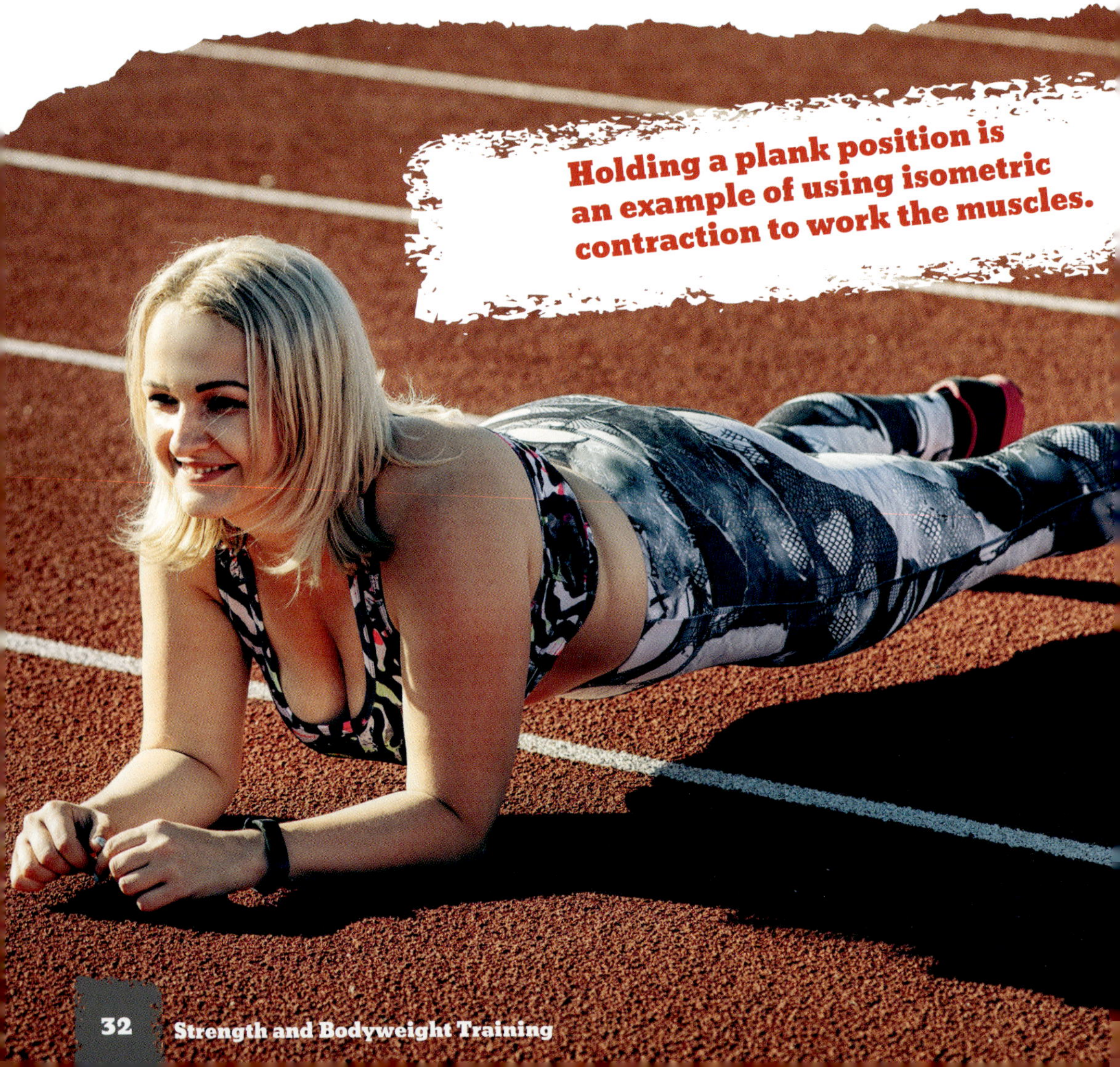

Holding a plank position is an example of using isometric contraction to work the muscles.

Strength and Bodyweight Training

Concentric

Concentric contraction involves a shortening of the muscle. Most common weightlifting exercises primarily focus on concentric contraction, such as a bicep curl. As your body pulls or pushes against the external force, the work is done to shorten the fibers through movement. Layers of actin and myosin slide across each other, ending up stacked closer together at the top. On lean, muscular bodies, this results in a visible bulge where the muscle contracts to its full extent.

Isometric

If you went outside and tried to pick up a car, it probably wouldn't move (unless you're one of the world's strongest people). However, if you really gave it your all in trying, you'd still leave panting, exhausted, and maybe even a bit sore. That's because isometric contraction still requires work.

Isometric literally means the same measurement, as in—if you measured the distance moved before and after the contraction, you wouldn't have gone anywhere. Isometric contractions, therefore, involve force production at the muscle without any movement of the limbs. Your muscle neither shortens nor lengthens, yet you're still working hard (think of holding a plank position or holding at the top of a pull-up).

Eccentric

Eccentric contraction involves resisting the lengthening of muscle fibers. Often, this requires a small concentric contraction first. Take a bicep curl for example—if you brought your wrist all the way to your shoulder without any resistance, the bicep would shorten. Yet if someone then grabbed your hand and tried to force it back down, against your resistance, you'd have to fight hard to win that battle. That's an eccentric contraction.

Some exercises, such as barbell squats and bench press, already set up the weight at the top of the movement. Therefore, you only have to resist the barbell as you descend to get an eccentric contraction.

BUILDING MUSCLE AND GETTING STRONGER

Consider what it takes to move through water on a boat. The harder you row, the more ripples you create. Similarly, the harder the muscle has to contract, the more metabolic damage it leaves behind. This is especially the case with eccentric contraction, given that the small "hooks" of actin and myosin are being ripped apart. To recover after a workout, your body shuttles nutrients and proteins to damaged areas, and it starts the rebuilding process.

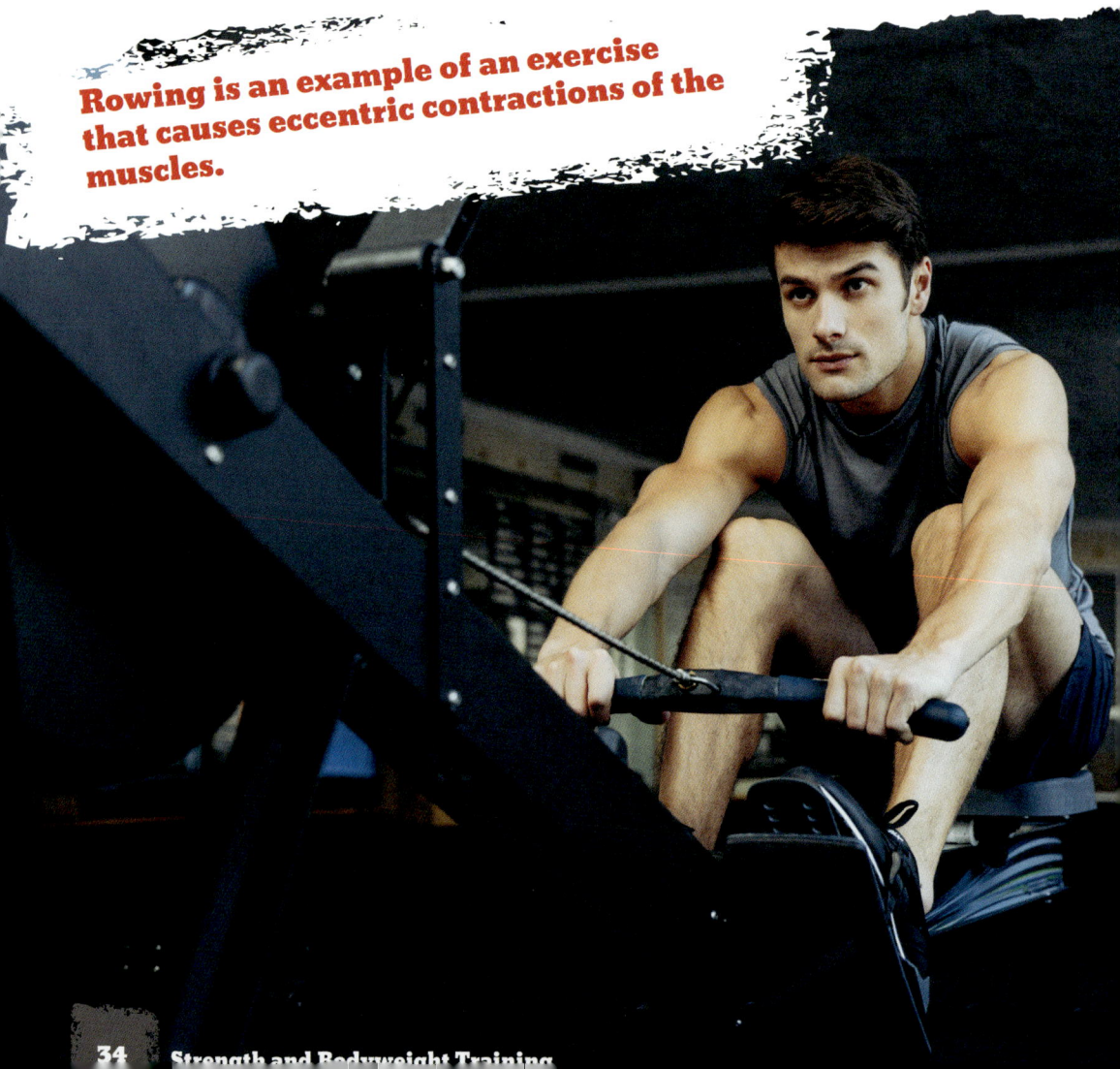

Rowing is an example of an exercise that causes eccentric contractions of the muscles.

When it comes to resistance training, our bodies build muscle through something known as the **SAID principle**, which stands for Specific Adaptation to Imposed Demands. This principle states that by placing an external demand on your body, it's forced to adapt accordingly. For example, doing a push-up challenges specific muscle fibers in your upper body to overcome resistance. To do so, your nerves signal movement, blood flows to that tissue, and mitochondria work overtime to create energy for contraction.

Hypertrophy

Hypertrophy, or the process of increasing muscle size, is triggered by three factors:

> Mechanical loading
> Metabolic stress
> Muscle damage

In their own individual ways, the above factors signal protein synthesis across the body. Therefore, it's possible to manipulate your strength training to build muscle size. However, none of it matters if you're not eating healthy and sleeping well, as that's when the real growth occurs.

Mechanical Loading

Whenever the body has to produce force to overcome an external

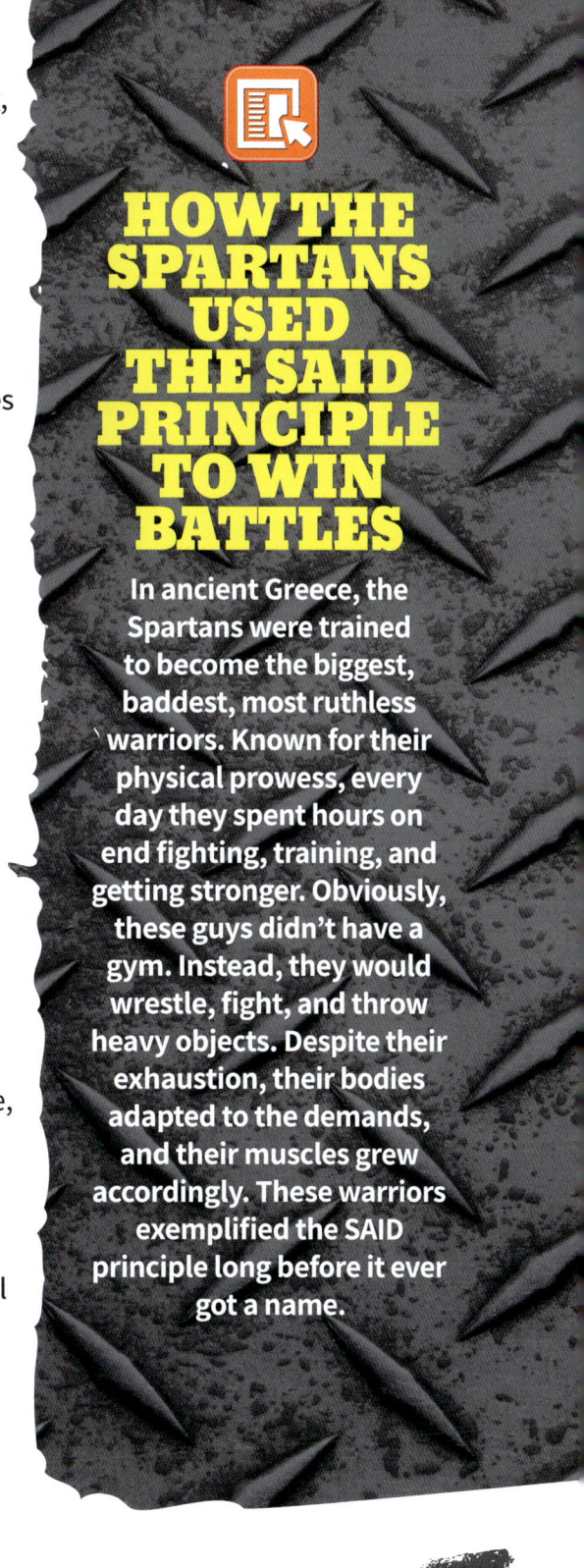

HOW THE SPARTANS USED THE SAID PRINCIPLE TO WIN BATTLES

In ancient Greece, the Spartans were trained to become the biggest, baddest, most ruthless warriors. Known for their physical prowess, every day they spent hours on end fighting, training, and getting stronger. Obviously, these guys didn't have a gym. Instead, they would wrestle, fight, and throw heavy objects. Despite their exhaustion, their bodies adapted to the demands, and their muscles grew accordingly. These warriors exemplified the SAID principle long before it ever got a name.

The Science Behind Resistance Training

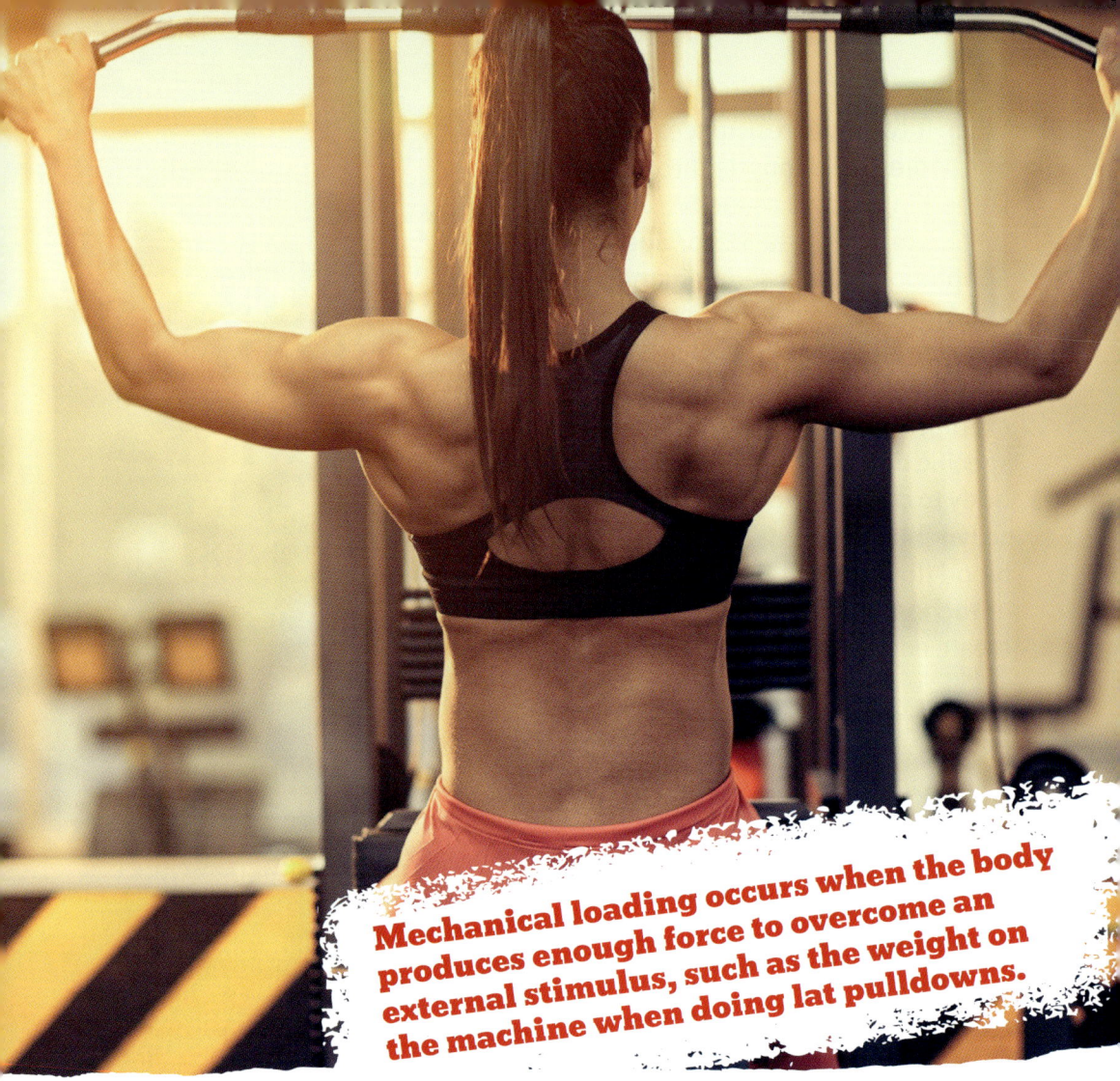

Mechanical loading occurs when the body produces enough force to overcome an external stimulus, such as the weight on the machine when doing lat pulldowns.

stimulus, that's mechanical loading. You could go outside and chop wood, climb a cliff, or deadlift boxes at work, but the easiest way to achieve this is by lifting weights. To increase a mechanical load, you either add weight, add reps, or increase the time under tension. In heavier sets, your body releases growth hormone, testosterone, and cortisol—three hormones that stimulate growth. Additionally, the more force you have to produce, the more motor units your muscles recruit.

Metabolic Stress

Metabolic stress involves your mitochondria, the little powerhouses within cells. These organelles work tirelessly to produce energy, especially during anaerobic metabolism. As strength training targets this energy system, it can be used to heavily stress your mitochondria. When these factories are overworked, your body creates more of them, relieving the pressure in expectation of further demands. As such, metabolic stress from resistance training increases mitochondrial density, which correlates with increased muscle size.

Muscle Damage

Finally, strength training can cause physical deformation of the muscle cell. Eccentric contraction is one of the best examples of this, as the actin

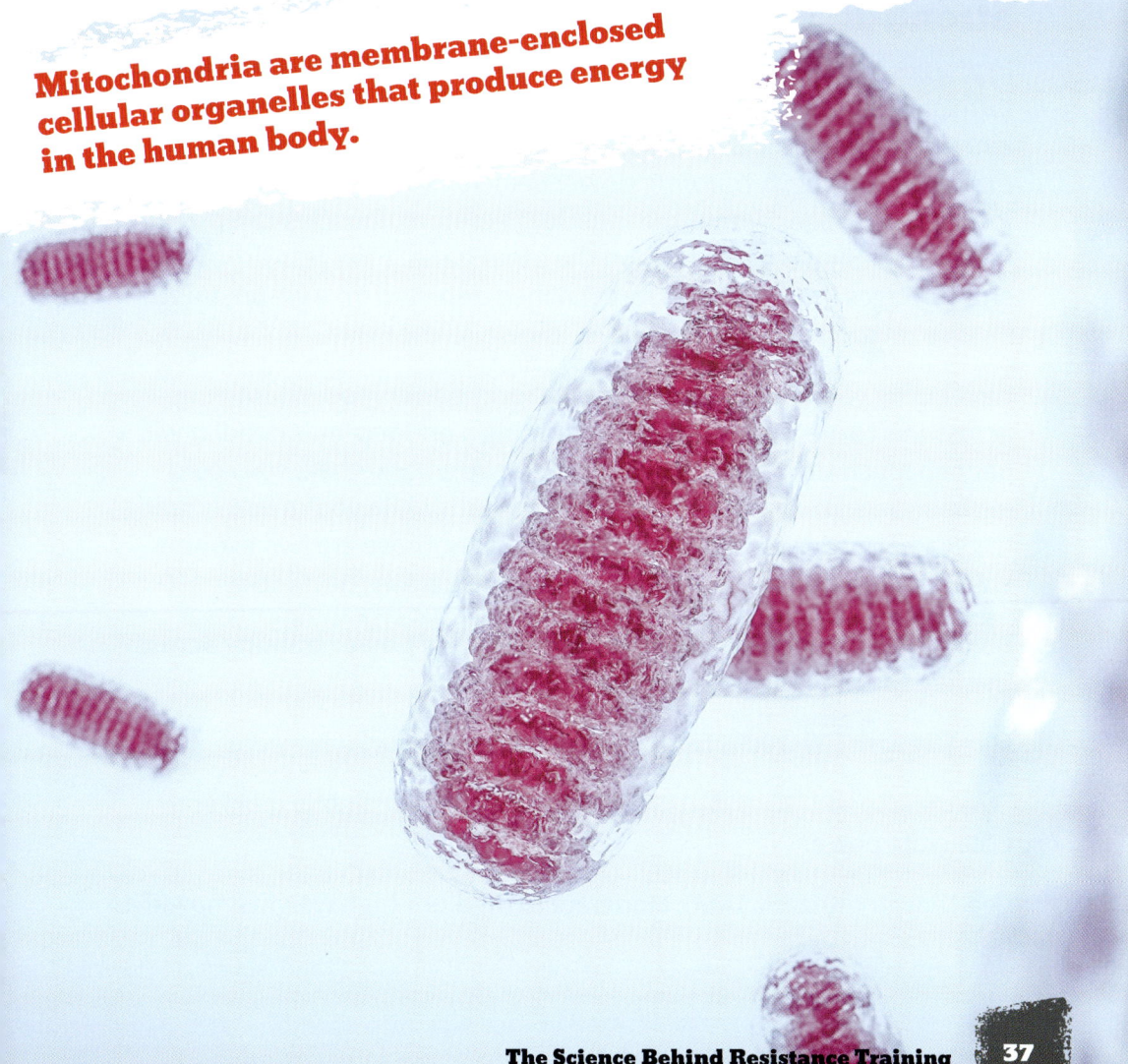

Mitochondria are membrane-enclosed cellular organelles that produce energy in the human body.

and myosin physically pull against each other, causing damage. Within myosin lie mechanosensors—small messengers that sense and respond to these changes.

As such, muscle damage triggers a whole cascade of events. The sensors release enzymes and transmitters that tell your body to start creating muscle protein. Think of it like an inspector noticing a hole in the wall. That inspector might call the building manager, who will call a contractor, who will gather all the materials needed to reinforce it. In order to avoid further damage, they'll make that area of the wall stronger than it was before. Your muscles, therefore, get bigger in response to the demands placed upon them.

Strength, Power, and Speed

In physics, power is the result of force times velocity. Thus, the two form an inverse relationship. As Penn State University professor of kinesiology Vladimir Zatsiorsky explains in his book *Science and Practice of Strength Training,* slower velocities allow for more time to form cross-bridges within the muscle. Therefore, muscles can produce more force. Higher velocities, on the other hand, offer less time for cross-bridges (and thus less force). When depicted on a graph, this inverse relationship forms a curve, known as the **force–velocity curve.**

Developing varying aspects of strength and power requires training across this curve. For example, performing a one-rep-max deadlift will happen much slower than simply picking up a basketball. You could probably even throw that ball over your head, while you're barely going to get a heavy deadlift to your hips. Obviously, those are two extreme ends, and most strength training lies somewhere in the middle.

Below is a basic guide describing strength and power training across the five zones of the force–velocity curve:

Max Strength (90–100% 1RM): Maximum force, slow movement

Strength–Speed (80–90% 1RM): High loads moved slightly quicker to accelerate power

Peak Power (30–80% 1RM): Moderate to medium-high weights moved as quickly as possible

Speed–Strength (30–60% 1RM): Less weight, geared toward developing velocity under load rather than outright power

Max Speed (<30% 1RM): Low or no loads, as fast as possible; best for training speed

Coordination

The human body has built-in systems to protect it from harm. One of these, the neuromuscular system, contains little mechanical neurons called proprioceptors that constantly provide feedback. They help ensure you can remain upright and not fall over. Bodyweight movements fine-tune these signals to make you incredibly adept at

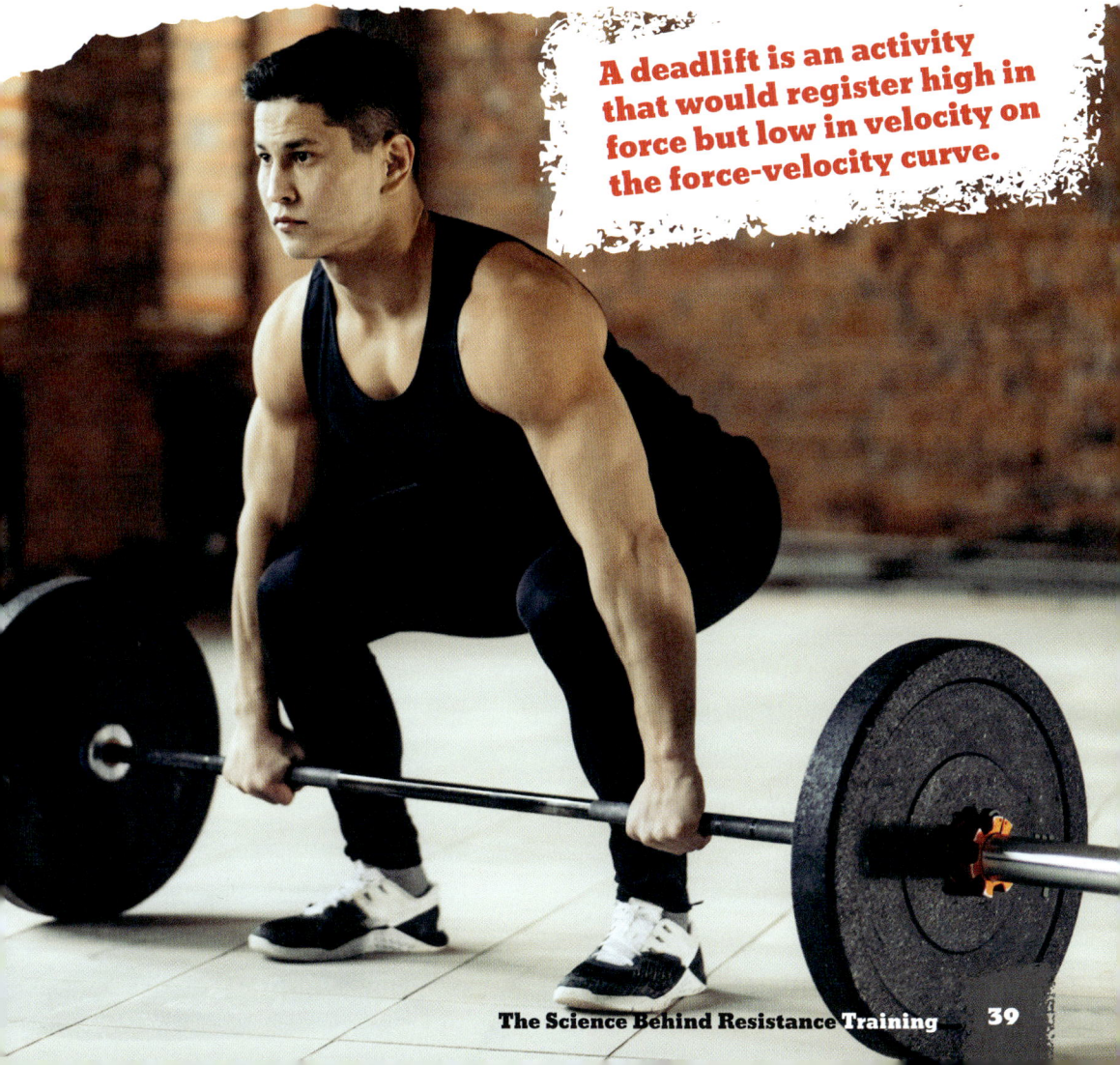

A deadlift is an activity that would register high in force but low in velocity on the force-velocity curve.

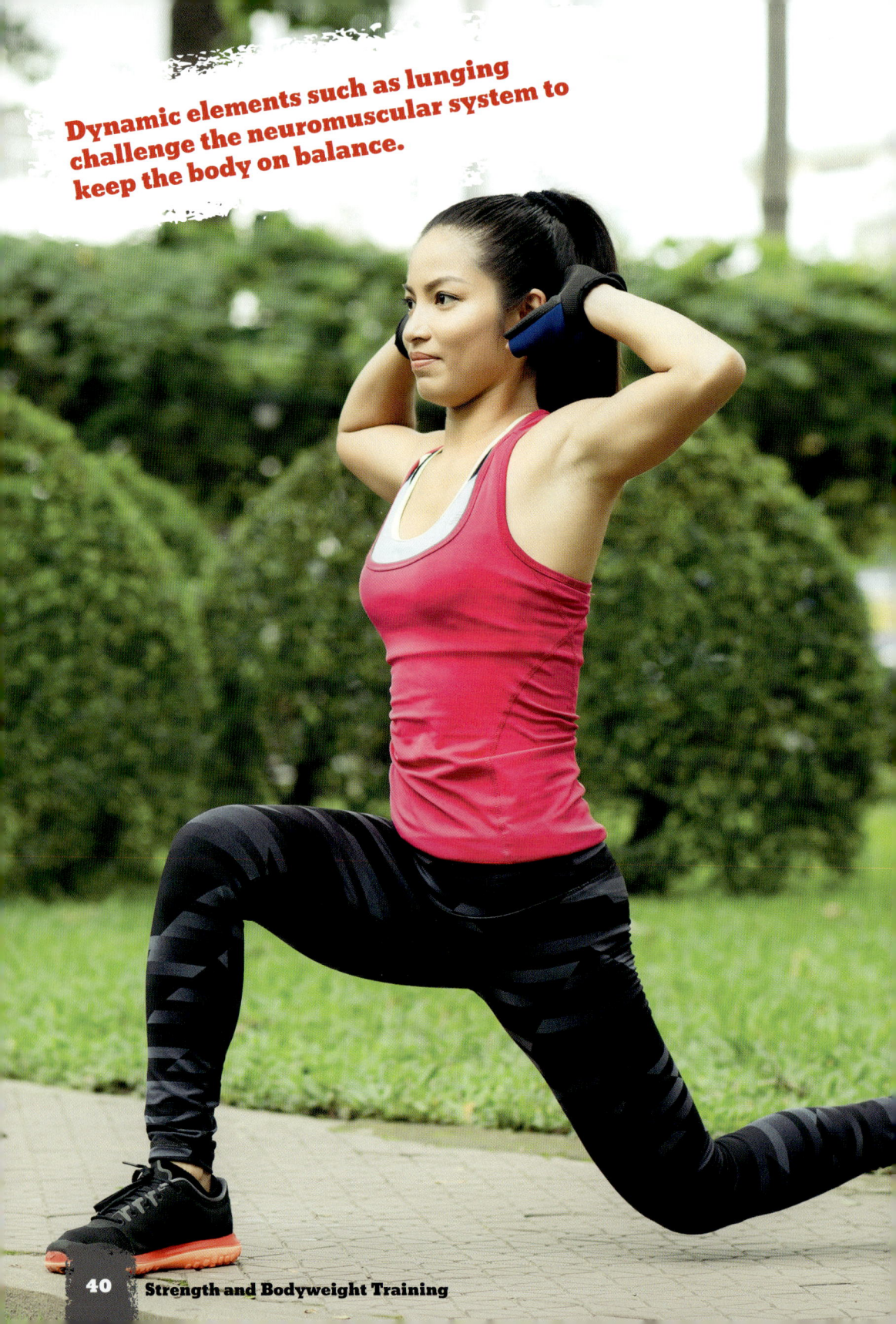

Dynamic elements such as lunging challenge the neuromuscular system to keep the body on balance.

reacting and staying balanced. The exception is in cases where the body predicts impending injury, and it involuntarily hinders strength and power output.

Coordination and practice allow the body to actually apply its strength and power in context. When we add a dynamic element, such as lunging, running, or cutting, this system gets challenged even further. With practice, however, our neuromuscular system learns efficient patterns.

Bodyweight training teaches our muscles the most efficient way to move, without even having to think about it. Therefore, you're free to run, jump, or play sports without having to worry about injury. Weight training allows adding an external load so that we can train our muscles to adapt, grow, and become athletic.

TEXT-DEPENDENT QUESTIONS

1. What percentage range of 1RM could you use to develop power?
2. Which type of muscle contraction results in the greatest mechanical muscle damage?
3. What is a motor unit, and how does it factor into muscle contraction?

RESEARCH PROJECT

People have been getting stronger since the dawn of time. It's only recently, however, that we've begun to understand how the human body works to build strength and muscle. For example, The First Congress for Scientific Research in Sport and Physical Exercise took place in Germany in 1912. Who were some of the other early adopters of exercise science? Research the history of the modern field of exercise science, and put together a short timeline of its growth into what it is today.

WORDS TO UNDERSTAND

density—the amount of work done over a specific period of time
intensity—the magnitude of difficulty in each repetition
repetition—a unit in weightlifting that represents a single instance of an exercise
set—a cluster of individual instances of an exercise that occur in succession
volume—the total amount of sets and repetitions completed

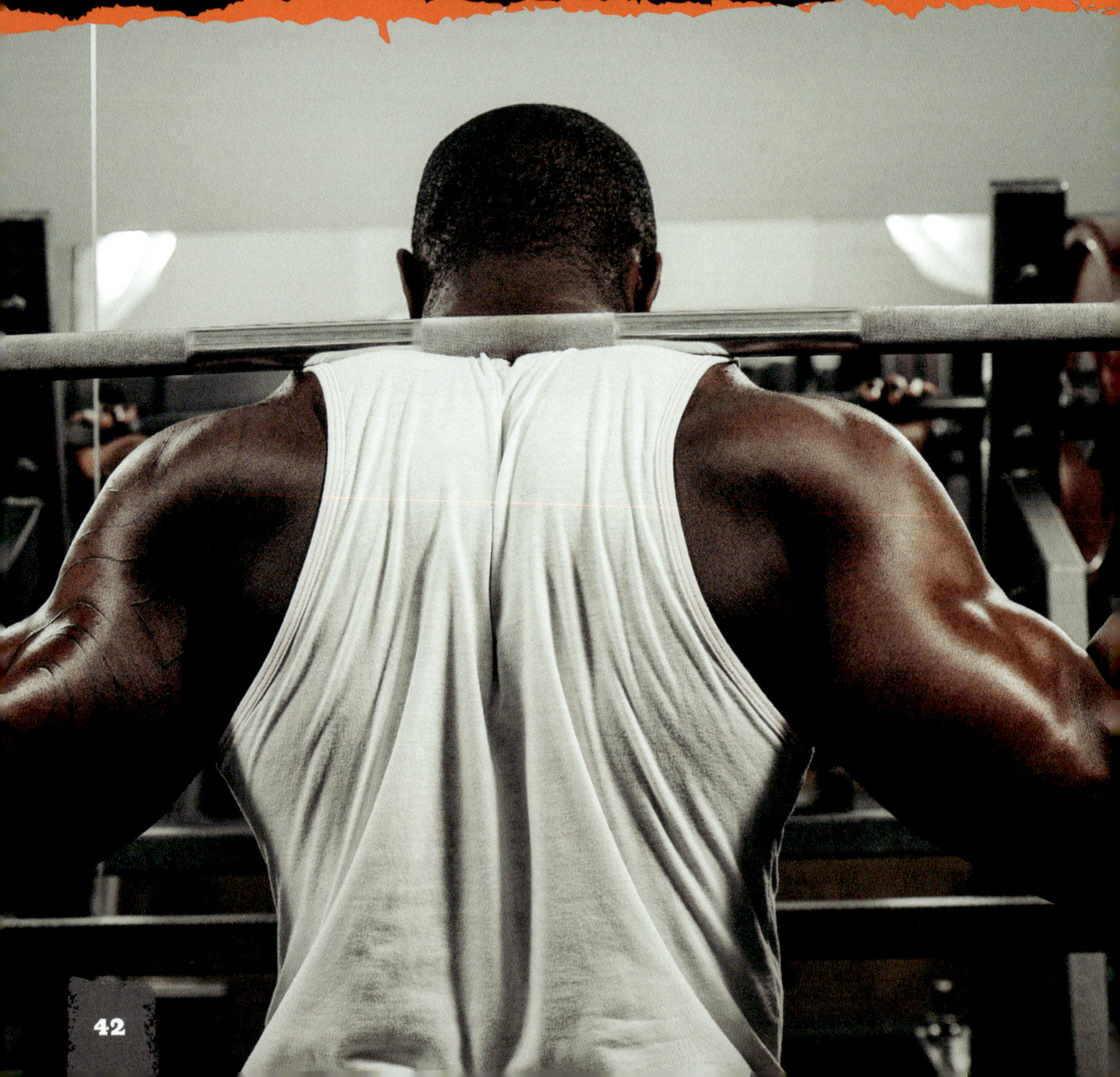

CHAPTER 4
BODYWEIGHT TRAINING VS. WEIGHT TRAINING

While we've talked a lot about bodyweight strength training, we haven't really touched on lifting weights. Although weight training is completely safe and highly beneficial for all populations, especially young people, you can't build a house without laying a strong foundation first. That's why bodyweight training serves as a solid starting point. Once you've mastered control of your own body, you can progress to weights.

Weight training involves external implements such as a barbell, dumbbells, or kettlebells. Obviously, this means you can lift more weight, as you're quite literally adding pounds. By doing so, you increase force production, challenge stability even further, and isolate greater ranges of motion.

Neither bodyweight training nor weight training is inherently better. Rather, they both offer unique benefits, and a well-rounded strength training program features both. Adding weight to a movement is a great way to make progress. By properly overloading your system with weights, you're likely to build muscle, get stronger, and perform better. As you get more advanced, bodyweight movements can sustain the mobility and stability required for daily activities, or you can manipulate it further for strength.

FACTORS TO CONSIDER

As previously mentioned, both bodyweight and weight training have their own advantages. Rather than simply choose one, it helps to think of the bigger picture. What are your goals? What equipment do you have access to? Are you just starting out, or have you been strength training for years? Finally, how can you manipulate your training session to achieve the desired results, regardless of the method?

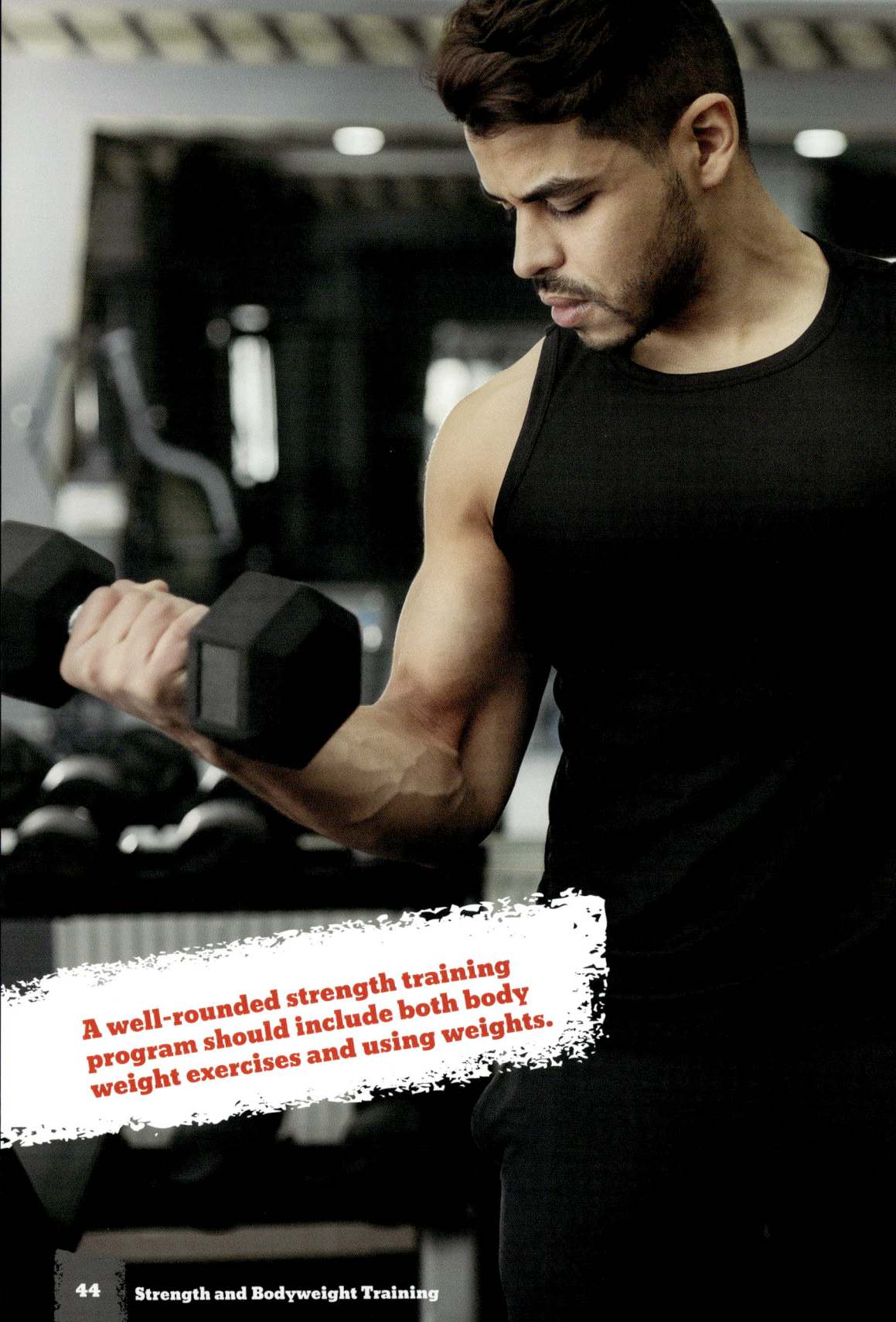

A well-rounded strength training program should include both body weight exercises and using weights.

When selecting your method of training, it's critical to understand how the following factors come into play:

> Repetitions
> Sets
> Volume
> Intensity
> Density

Through careful manipulation of these factors, you can achieve a lot of strength training goals with both bodyweight and weight training.

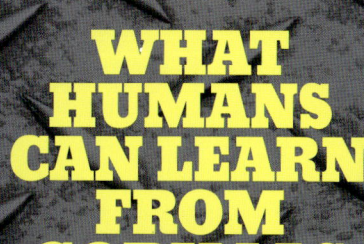

WHAT HUMANS CAN LEARN FROM GORILLAS

Gorillas, like humans, are primates—and incredibly strong ones at that. How do they get that way? Part of it is genetics, of course, but part of it is bodyweight training. While gorillas don't hit the gym, they regularly climb, knuckle-walk, and push and pull their weight around. This helps build and maintain functional muscle. Fortunately, humans don't have to brave the wilderness to survive, but that doesn't mean we can't borrow some guerrilla tactics to build strength.

A woman does reps of weighted squats. If she does multiple groups of reps, those are referred to as sets.

 Manipulating intensity and volume is important in resistance training. This video shows you why.

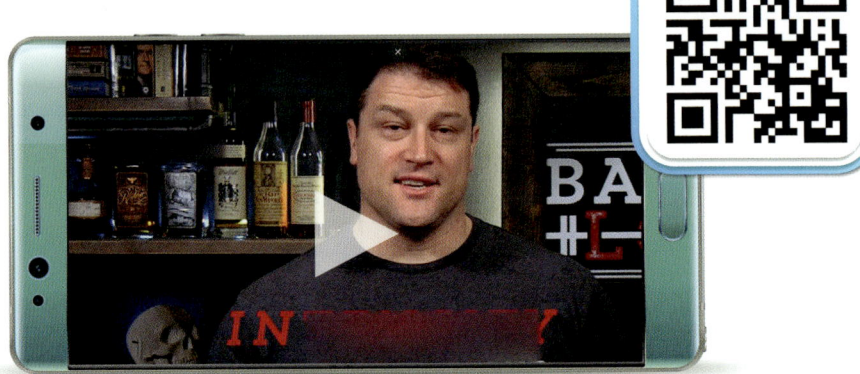

A **repetition**, or rep, is a single instance of an exercise. If you did 10 squats, that equals 10 reps. **Sets** are groups of repetitions. If you repeated those 10 squats after a period of rest, that would represent 2 sets of 10 reps. Sets and reps are the backbones of resistance training. Every single program works around these two basic building blocks. In general, they have an inverse relationship. The more reps you do, the fewer sets you can complete, and vice versa.

Volume, on the other hand, is the total number of reps and sets of an exercise you complete in a session. Whether you do 3 sets of 10 (3 x 10) or 10 sets of 3 (10 x 3), that still equals a total volume of 30. In contrast, **intensity** measures the difficulty of each individual rep. You can make a rep more intense by adding weight, lengthening time under tension, increasing the velocity, or adjusting the impact of gravity. For example, to make a bodyweight squat more intense, you might do a jump squat instead. You could also add weight, hold it for 10 seconds at the bottom, or do it on one leg.

Finally, **density** refers to the amount of work you can complete in a certain amount of time. A workout becomes denser the faster you can complete a certain volume and intensity of work. Doing 30 total reps in 5 minutes, therefore, is denser than a volume of 30 reps in 30 minutes. Increasing density is a great way to add difficulty to bodyweight exercises especially, as you can't just pick up a heavier body weight from the rack.

HOW TO USE BODYWEIGHT AND WEIGHT TRAINING TO REACH YOUR GOALS

Now that we've gone over the factors at play during both methods of resistance training, how can you apply them to your workouts? Let's look at a few common goals of strength training to figure it out.

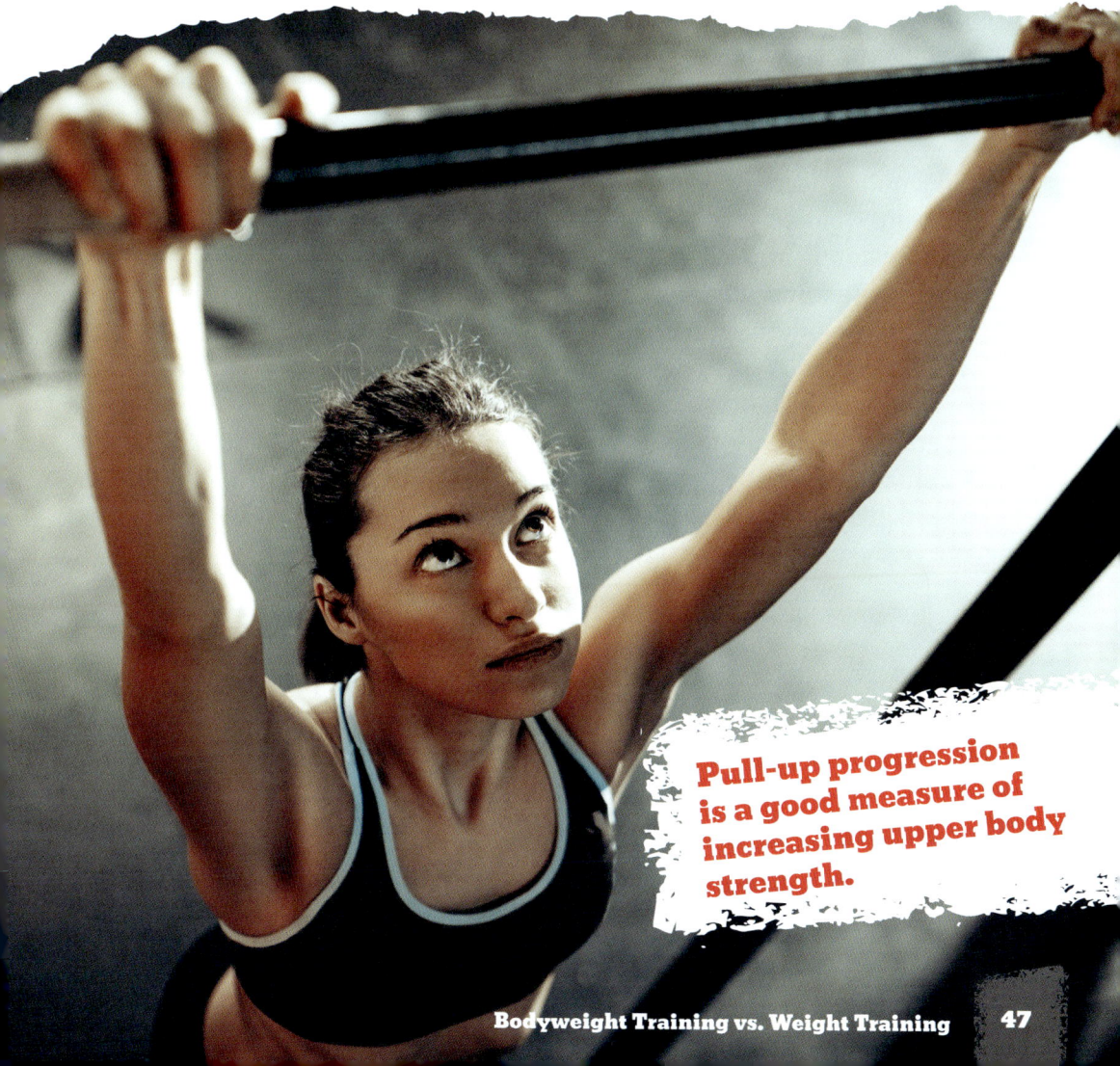

Pull-up progression is a good measure of increasing upper body strength.

Training for Maximum Strength

To increase strength, you need to add intensity to your workouts. If you remember, this can be accomplished by adding load, velocity, time, or adjusting for gravity.

Get Strong Using Your Own Body Weight

"You can't get stronger with bodyweight training."

The above statement is a common misconception. Let's consider the pull-up as an example. If you start out not being able to complete one pull-up, and you work toward a single rep, have you gotten stronger? Yes! You can now complete a movement that requires more upper body strength. Likewise, being able to do three, four, or five pull-ups would indicate a progression in strength. Someone who can do a single-arm pull-up is significantly stronger than someone who can't do one with both arms, given the same body weight.

As you'll notice from the above example, increasing the load with bodyweight training required manipulating the effect of gravity. While gravity constantly applies the same force upon us, physics dictates that we can move a force with more ease (or greater difficulty, in this case) by changing lever lengths and angles in relation to the fulcrum. Your body works like a complex set of levers and pulleys, and you can put yourself at a mechanical advantage or disadvantage by adjusting your position. In general, the more of your body weight that you move against gravity with a smaller lever, the harder it will be. That's why a single-arm pull-up is so hard. It's one small lever (one arm) moving a lot of weight (the rest of your body) directly against gravity (straight up).

That's just one example. You could also add static holds to an exercise, or even increase the velocity in some cases. Overall, use your body weight to get stronger by first adding reps to an exercise you can do comfortably, then change the effect of gravity, manipulate the tempo, and repeat as needed.

Resistance Training for Strength

While there are multiple ways to train for strength, the oldest and most popular method is the percentage of one-rep maximum. This is done

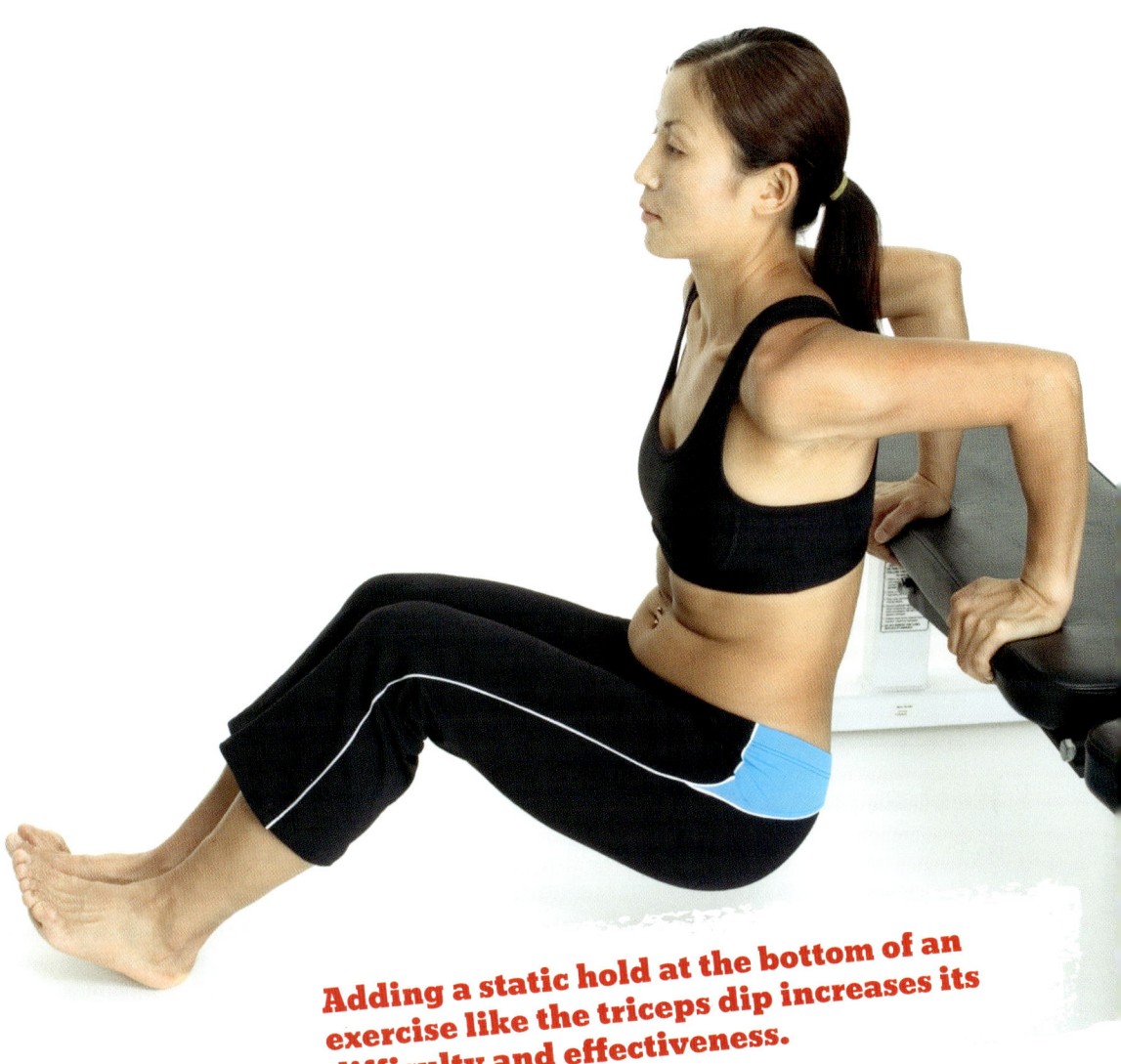

Adding a static hold at the bottom of an exercise like the triceps dip increases its difficulty and effectiveness.

by calculating the heaviest weight you can lift in a movement, such as a squat, and lifting a certain percentage of it for a prescribed amount of repetitions and sets. Despite some concerns, one-repetition max testing is safe and effective when done correctly. Always make sure to adequately prepare the body to lift maximal loads before even coming close to attempting it. It's recommended that anyone new to testing do so under the supervision of a trained professional.

Once you've determined your one-rep max for a given exercise, it's time to get to work. Thanks to a Soviet weightlifting coach from the 1970s and

1980s, Alexander Sergeyevitch Prilepin, we have a chart bearing his name for calculation. Prilepin's Chart, featured below, shows the ideal amount of sets and reps of an exercise to perform at a certain percentage to yield maximum strength. For example, a newer weightlifter might want to start on the lower end of total range. Therefore, they might choose to train with 4 sets of 6 reps at 60% of their one-rep max. As the weeks pass, and that lifter gets stronger, they could progress to 5 sets of 5 at 65%, then 6 sets of 3 at 75%, and so on. Years of research in the lab and the gym have proven this a highly effective training method for developing starting strength.

Prilepin's Chart

Percent	Reps/Sets	Optimal	Total Range
55–65	3–6	24	18–30
70–80	3–6	18	12–24
80–90	2–4	15	10–20
90+	1–2	4	10

Resistance Training to Build Muscle

Weight training is the clear winner in this category. While not impossible to put on size with bodyweight training, it takes a lot of time, a lot of food, and a lot of expertise. Research has shown that training multiple sets of somewhere between 6–12 concentric reps at the heaviest weight you can maintain induces hypertrophy. There are also strong cases for eccentric and isometric training methods. Others focus more on shorter rest periods. The truth is, there's no ONE way to build muscle, but it does seem that lifting weights gets you there much faster.

When training for hypertrophy, you should focus primarily on large, multi-joint movements such as squats, deadlifts, bench press, overhead press, pull-ups, and rows. Accessory movements should follow to target specific areas, such as leg extensions for the quadriceps or tricep extensions for the triceps.

Resistance Training for Speed

If you want to get fast, you've got to sprint. Technically, sprinting is a sequence of plyometric exercises—just one single leg bound after the next. Therefore, practicing bodyweight plyometrics can get you faster. Learning the mechanics of jumping, landing, and stopping will make you more energy efficient as you go to sprint. Not only that, but it'll train your motor units to work at a high intensity. With continued training, your central nervous system starts to pick up on the demands of plyometrics, and your neuromuscular system adapts.

Despite just using your body weight, plyometrics constitute maximal effort exercises every time. As such, they should be incorporated into training accordingly, especially at the youth level. Aim for one plyometric session per week at the start to avoid injury and try to keep the total volume down. According to *Plyometrics*, by Donald A. Chu and Gregory

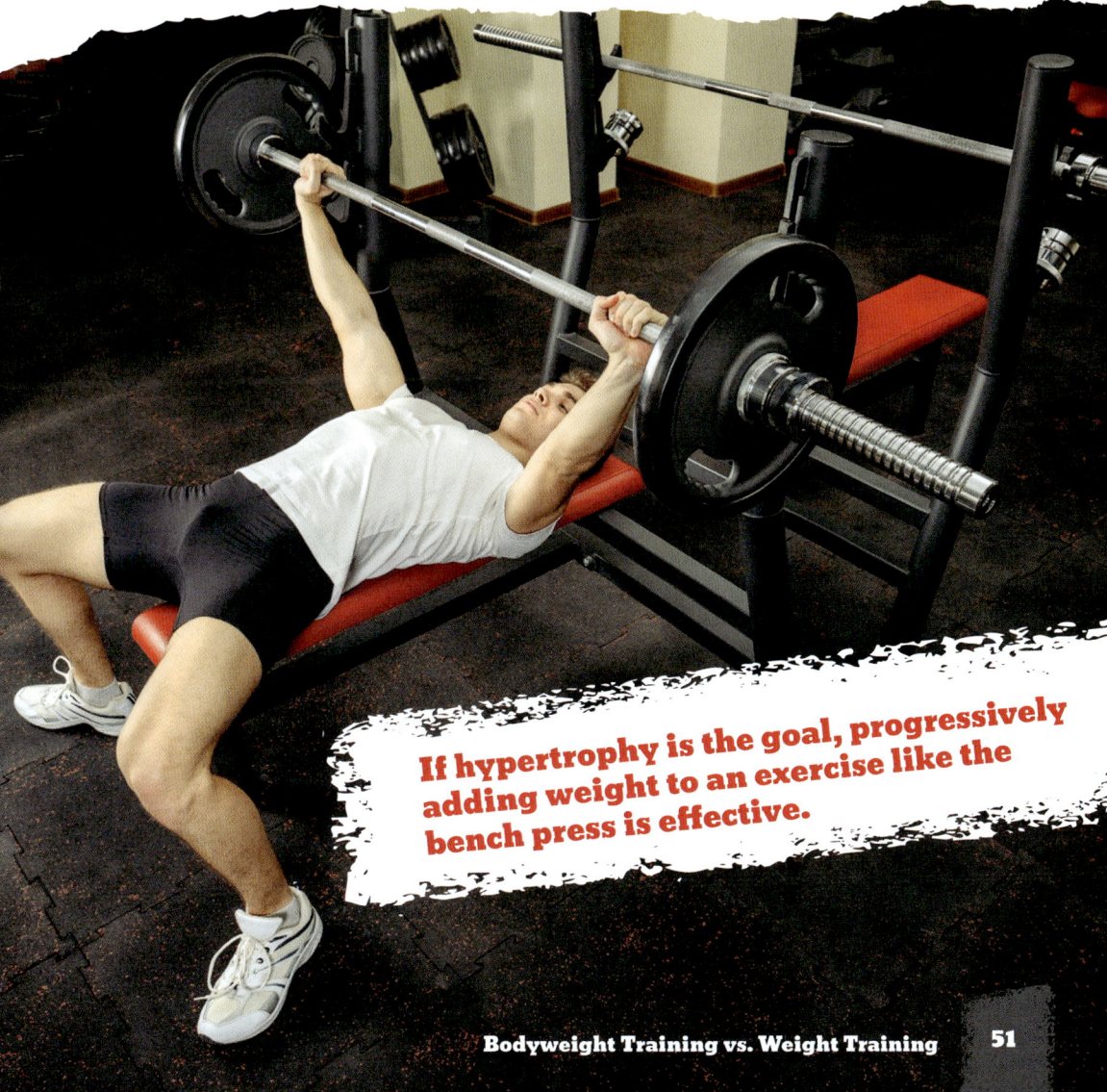

If hypertrophy is the goal, progressively adding weight to an exercise like the bench press is effective.

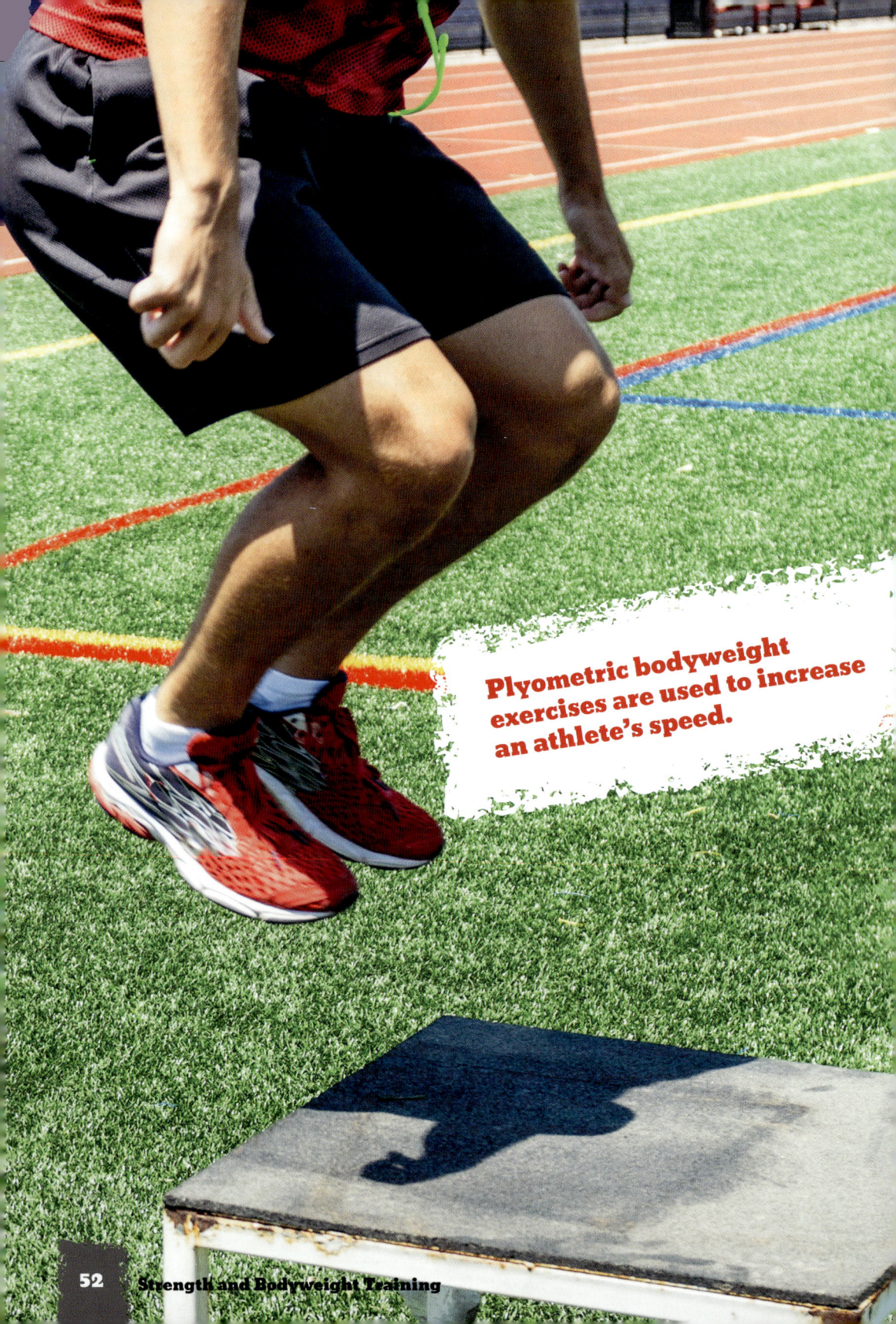

Plyometric bodyweight exercises are used to increase an athlete's speed.

Meyer, "guidelines for volume prescription related to a single plyometric training bout based on experience level suggest that adult athletes with novice experience should employ a training volume with 80 to 100 foot contacts per session while adult athletes with more experience can use 120 to 140 foot contacts per session."

Weight Training for Speed

When using weights to develop speed, it's crucial to employ lighter weights that allow for explosive movements. Hang cleans, kettlebell swings, and weighted jumps are great lower body activities, while medicine ball throws and explosive rows help the upper body. Despite going for maximum velocity, proper form is paramount to avoid injury. Never attempt a weight you can't perform comfortably at speed.

TEXT-DEPENDENT QUESTIONS

1. Name the five factors that are manipulated to achieve strength training goals.
2. What are the benefits of bodyweight training for speed?
3. Name three ways to increase the intensity of a workout both with and without using weights.

RESEARCH PROJECT

There are few places bodyweight and weight training collide like Muscle Beach in Venice, CA. This iconic beach features an outdoor gym, complete with equipment designed for calisthenics and heavy weights. All year long, people flock to Muscle Beach to show off their strength. Research Muscle Beach workouts and find 3–4 videos of weight training workouts to compare and contrast with bodyweight workouts. What techniques do they use? How do they train the same muscle groups differently? Which do you prefer?

WORDS TO UNDERSTAND

long-term athlete development—a seven-stage model for developing athletes from infancy to adulthood, originally coined by Istvan Balyi

peak height velocity—the period during maturation when a child experiences his or her fastest upward growth; also marking a critical period for the onset of periodized strength training

vectors—objects with both a magnitude and direction, such as a certain amount of directed force

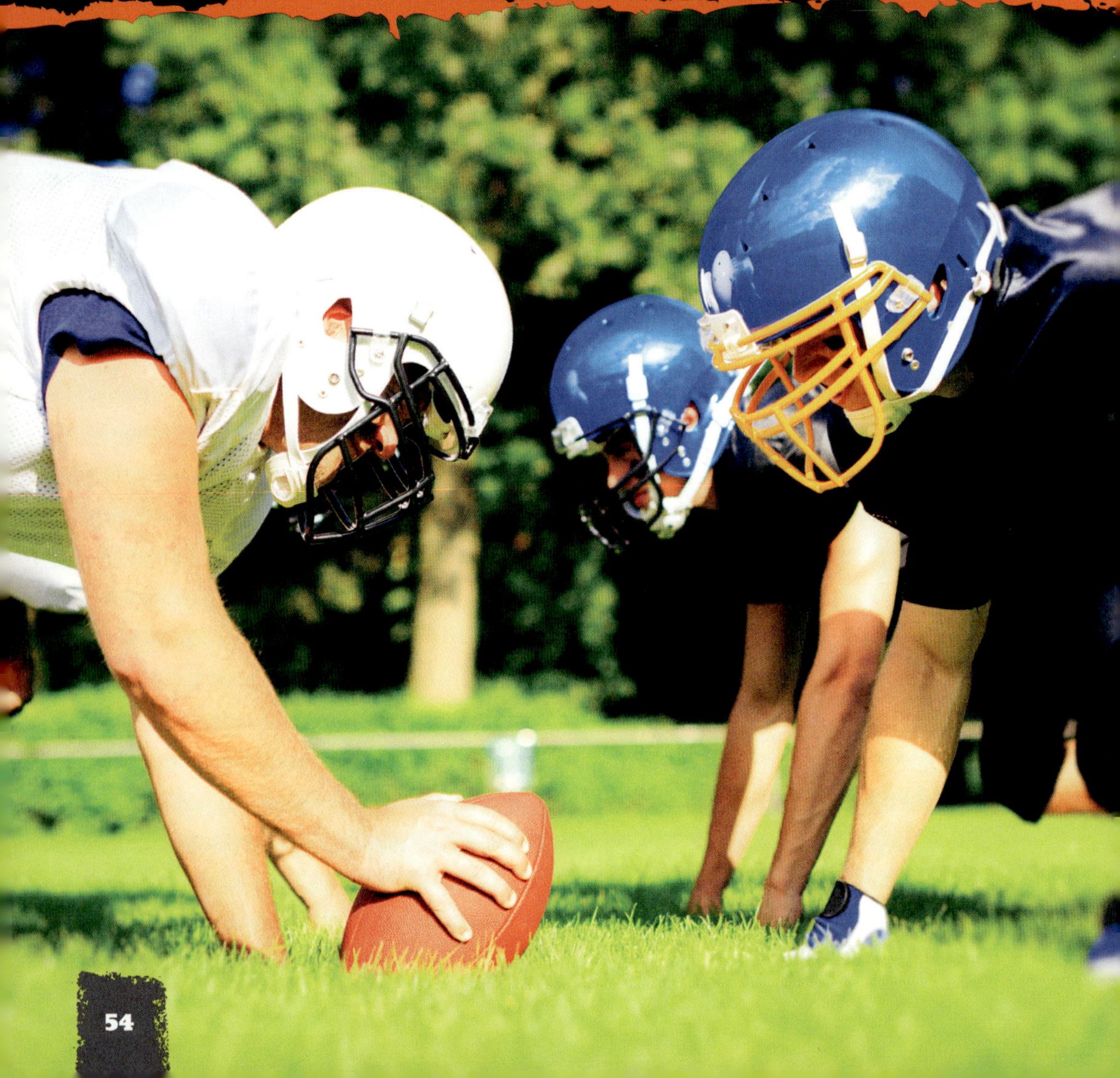

CHAPTER 5
STRENGTH TRAINING FOR YOUNG ATHLETES

As an athlete, strength training is the first line of defense against injury. Sports involve repetitive, maximal effort movements that place a ton of stress on muscles, bones, ligaments, and tendons. Strength training not only protects those tissues, but it can even make them stronger and more powerful than those of the opponent.

In order to perform on game day, you have to prepare! Just like you wouldn't show up to a game without practicing your skills, it's a bad idea go into a competition without physical preparation either.

THE BENEFITS OF STRENGTH TRAINING FOR ATHLETIC PERFORMANCE

Young athletes have the most to gain from strength training, as it directly translates to performance in competition. Greater strength means the ability to produce more force, which correlates with speed and power. Improved biomechanics groove neuromuscular patterns, so you don't have to think twice about cutting, tackling, or jumping. Training stability through a full range of motion can prevent injury, and target strengthening of certain muscles balances the strain placed on the body from repetitive activity. Finally, it helps to build confidence to overcome obstacles and achieve goals.

In general, young athletes can expect the following benefits from proper strength training:

> Injury prevention
> Increased force production
> Speed improvement

- > Better coordination
- > Improved balance
- > Reduced fatigue in competition and practice
- > Increased mood, confidence, and sense of self-efficacy

However, every athlete is an individual and should be treated as such. One of the major factors in strength training for young athletes is their long-term development. Specialization and emphasis on performance too early can be a detriment to success, contributing to injury and burnout. Therefore, in 1995, a sport scientist named Istvan Balyi came up with a four-stage **Long-Term Athlete Development** (LTAD) model that has since grown to the following seven stages.

LONG-TERM ATHLETE DEVELOPMENT

Stage 1: Active Start (0-6 Years of Age)

At this stage, it's all about learning to move well. You're still adapting to crawling, walking, climbing, and running. Kids at this stage need to stay active every day and explore how their bodies can interact with the

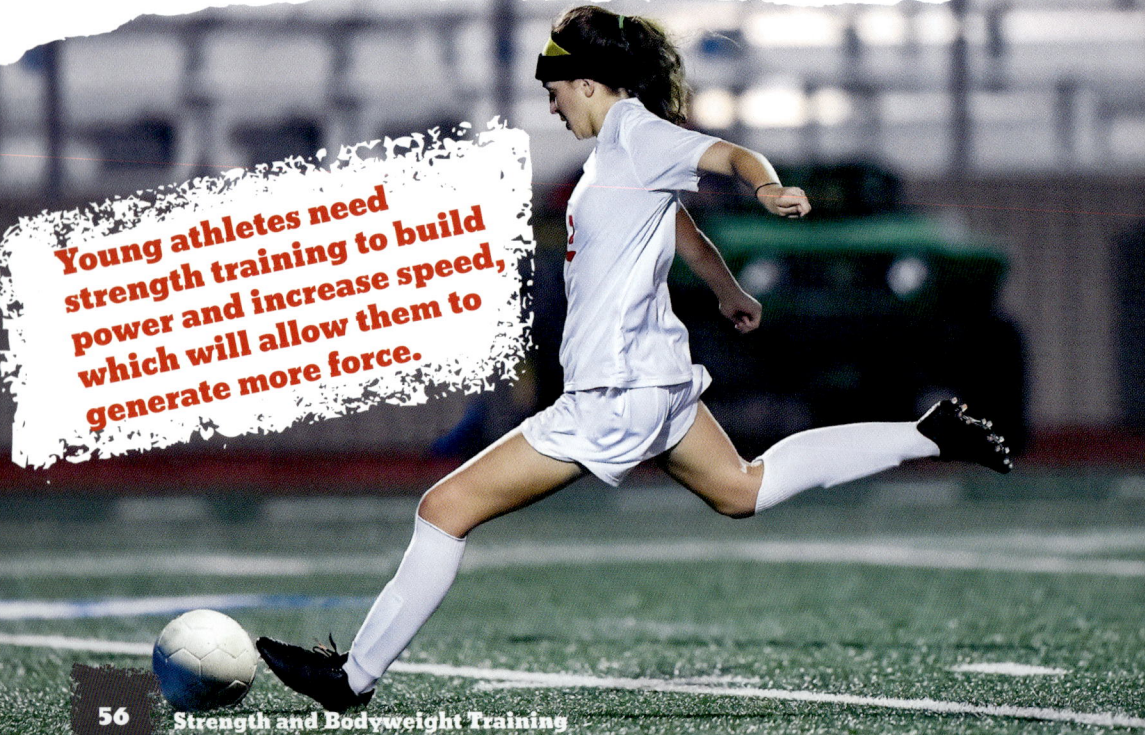

Young athletes need strength training to build power and increase speed, which will allow them to generate more force.

environment. Sure, some young kids may start playing a sport during this stage, but it's all about play.

Stage 2: Fundamentals (0-9 Years in Boys, 0-8 Years in Girls)

Still all about having fun, children in stage 2 of development might start to refine some of those movement skills they learned earlier. Athletic activity becomes more structured, such as joining youth sports leagues, but the focus remains heavily on having fun. Basic bodyweight exercises can be taught, but avoid a fully structured strength program.

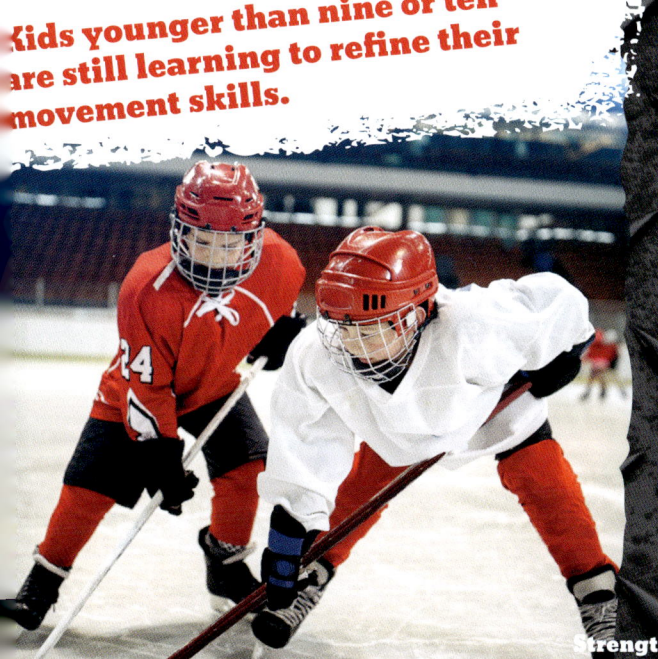

Kids younger than nine or ten are still learning to refine their movement skills.

WHEN YOU PEAK TOO YOUNG: USING LTAD TO ADDRESS BURNOUT

When working with Canadian national teams, Istvan Balyi noticed a trend. Athletes started off strong, but the grueling training sessions caught up with them. While they won in the short-term, Team Canada was losing its best athletes to injury and burnout before their prime. Calling upon the famous "10,000 hour rule," Balyi decided to change that. Research had proven that it takes 8–12 years to become truly elite, so he created the LTAD model as a framework for success. Now his work is used by coaches worldwide to win national and international championships.

Stage 3: Learn to Train (From Ages 8-9 Until Hitting the Growth Spurt Around 10-11 Years of Age)

During this stage, children should start developing foundational sport skills. In the case of weight training, this means either fine-tuning or introducing bodyweight exercises such as push-ups, pull-ups, squats, lunges, and planks. Avoid the temptation to specialize in one sport by utilizing strength training to develop proficiency in a variety of athletic skills.

Stage 4: Train to Train (After the Onset of the Growth Spurt, Usually Around 11-15 Years for Girls or 12-16 Years for Boys)

Everyone's growth spurt happens at a different time, but once it starts, it marks a time in which young athletes can feasibly begin a strength training program. In exercise science, this is known as your **peak height velocity**. Therefore, you'll start applying the information learned in this book during this stage. The main focus remains the development of skills and movement foundation, but you can start to include some performance outcomes.

Stage 5: Train to Compete (16-23 Years in Boys , 15-21 Years in Girls)

This is the final stage of youth training, as you're aging into adulthood during this period. When training to compete, athletes are regularly involved in structured practices and competitions, and many will begin to specialize in one specific sport. The goal, as indicated by the name, is to develop your existing strengths to be able to compete with other athletes of the same age and experience level. Athletes will begin implementing weight training regularly as a part of this goal and should be involved in a structured, progressive, and well-thought-out strength training program.

Stages 6 & 7: Train to Win and Active for Life

Athletes may transition into the "Train to Win" stage if they turn professional. In this environment, world-class competition, facilities,

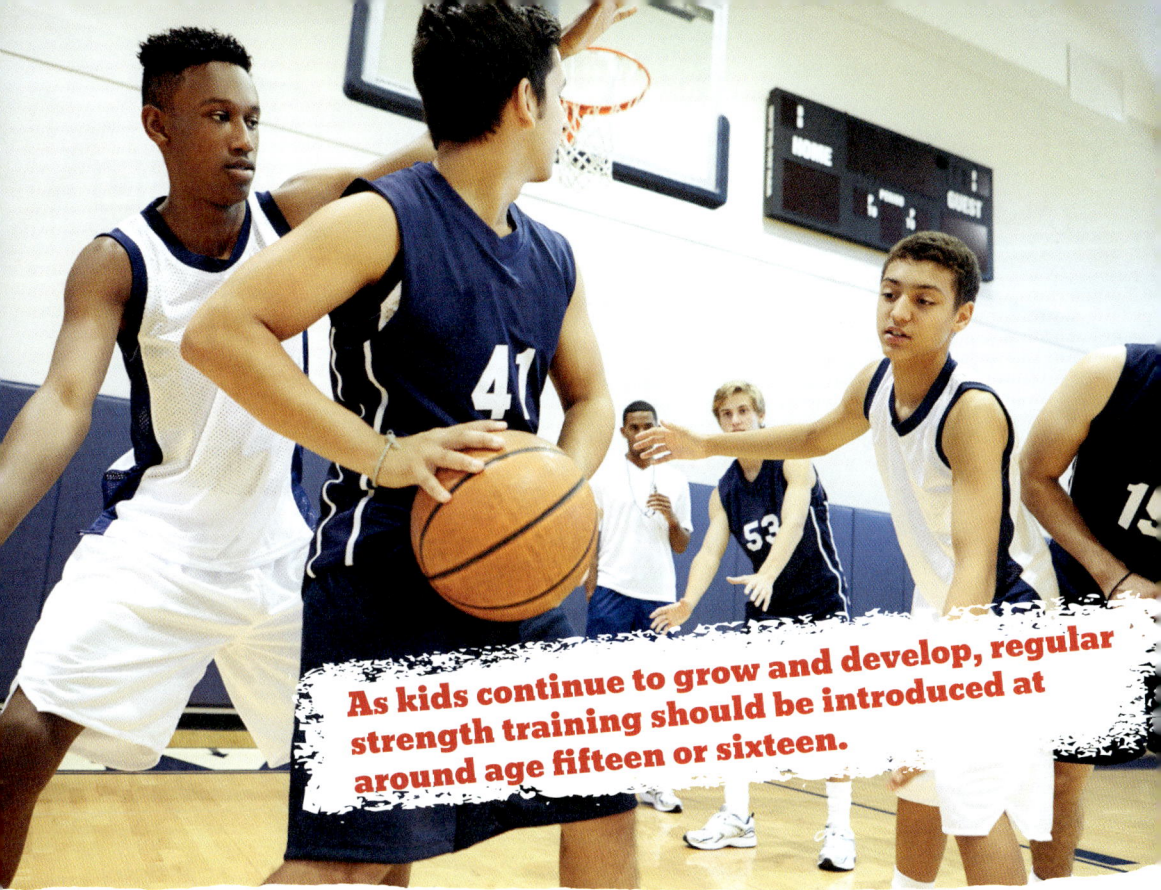

As kids continue to grow and develop, regular strength training should be introduced at around age fifteen or sixteen.

and management are required to match the demands of a high-intensity professional schedule year-round. After the completion of their careers, athletes become active for life, maintaining a healthy balance of strength training to promote overall well-being. The "Active for Life" stage covers all ages, as some athletes may never want to pursue competitive sports. In this case, they simply use strength training as a tool to stay healthy.

DEVELOPING A STRENGTH PLAN FOR YOUNG ATHLETES

For this book, we're going to focus on Stages 4 and 5 of the Long-Term Athlete Development model, from preteen years to early adulthood.

 Watch professional sports trainers talk about strength training for youth athletes.

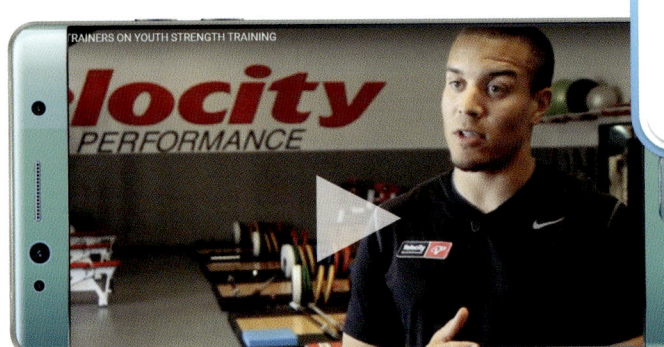

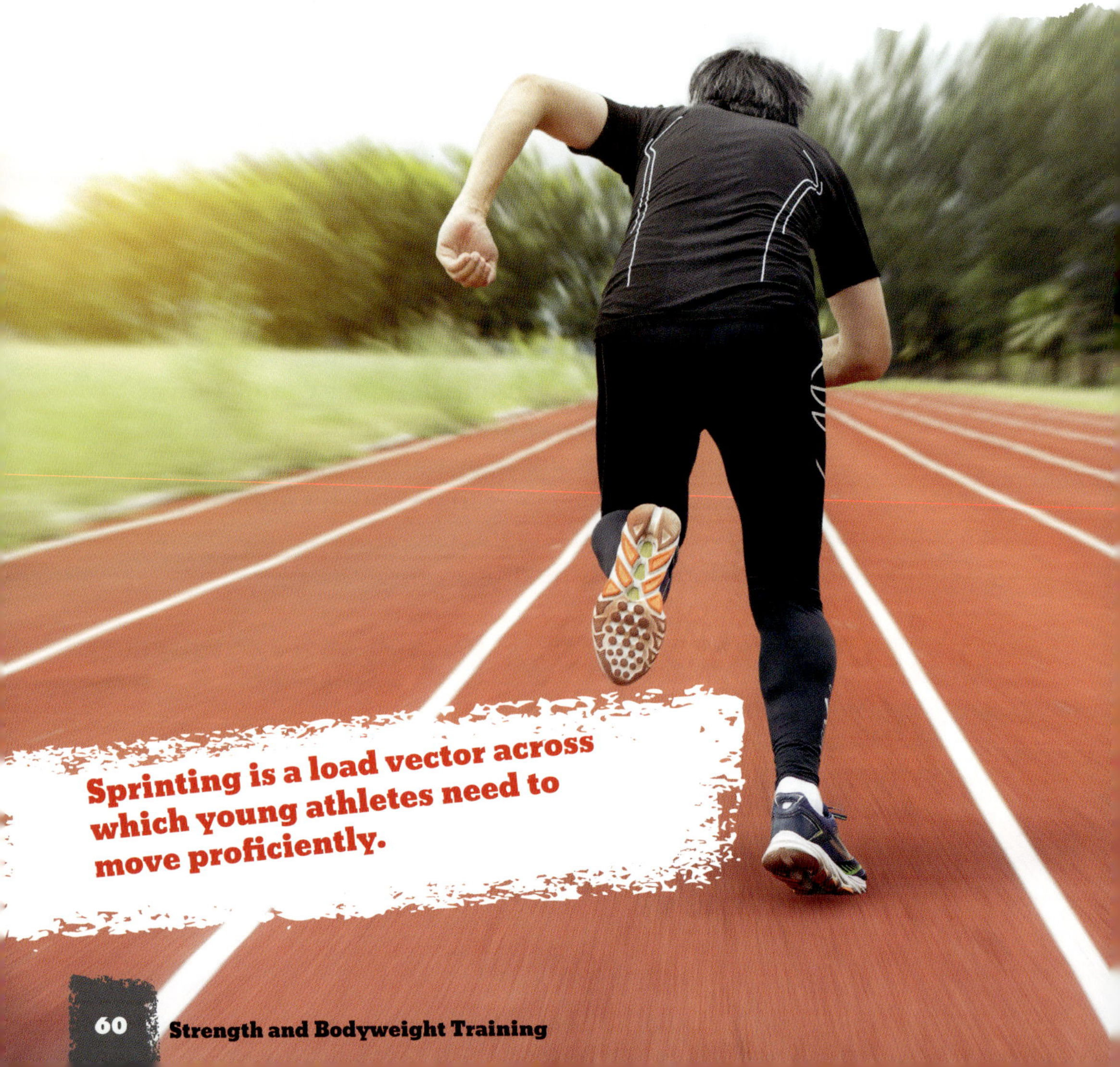

Sprinting is a load vector across which young athletes need to move proficiently.

Keep It Simple

You might see some athletes doing impressive, fancy tricks on social media. Despite looking cool, there's no need to attempt to overcomplicate your training. Focus on the fundamentals and build a strength foundation before anything else. In sports, young athletes need to move proficiently across the following load **vectors**:

1. Vertical jumping
2. Horizontal acceleration
3. Top-speed sprinting
4. Cutting/lateral running
5. Deceleration/Backpedaling
6. Twisting

Accordingly, weight training can be used to train those dynamics. Plyometrics, for instance, represent carefully programmed practices of all of the above. Furthermore, other resistance training can be modified to build strength, stability, power, and coordination while managing the total load to avoid injury. Therefore, weight training programs for young athletes should include the following movements:

1. Upper body push
2. Upper body pull
3. Lower body quad dominant
4. Lower body hip dominant
5. Rotational
6. Carrying

Overall, a strength training program for young athletes should target the major muscle groups equally across the entire body. While certain sports might focus on a specific area—soccer players might train legs while baseball players might need more upper body—follow the general guidelines above to develop a well-rounded athlete.

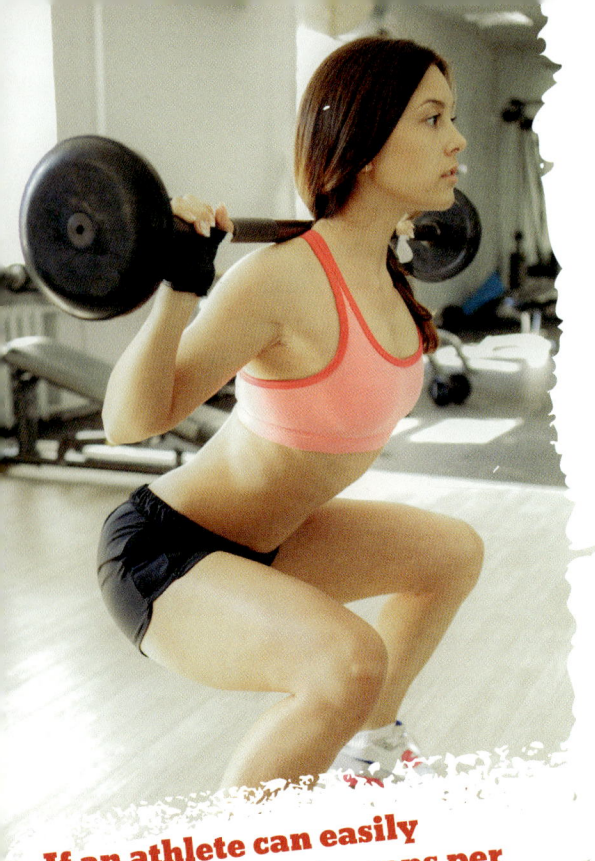

SETS, REPS, AND PROGRESSION

Young athletes will begin training with 1–3 sets of 10–20 repetitions of each exercise at a weight they can manage with proper form. But how do you know when it's time to progress? An easy guideline to follow—once you can easily complete two more reps more than prescribed on every set for 2 weeks, it's time to change something. Progression can mean adding more weight, increasing reps, adding even more weight and decreasing reps, changing position, or manipulating speed.

If an athlete can easily complete two extra reps per set for 2 weeks, she should increase the weight, number of reps, or speed in each set.

For specific performance goals, here are Prilepin's Chart and the force-velocity curve again, which were previously referenced in earlier chapters:

Prilepin's Chart for Strength Training

Prilepin's Chart

Percent	Reps/sets	Optimal	Total Range
55–65	3–6	24	18–30
70–80	3–6	18	12–24
80–90	2–4	15	10–20
90+	1–2	4	10

The Force-Velocity Curve

Max Strength (90–100% 1RM)

Strength-Speed (80–90% 1RM)

Peak Power (30–80% 1RM)

Speed-Strength (30–60% 1RM)

Max Speed (<30% 1RM)

As you can see, lower rep ranges correlate with higher intensities and vice versa. When training for speed and power, the lighter the weight, the faster you can move it. Use anywhere from 1–6 reps for maximum strength, speed, and power, move to 6–12 reps for hypertrophy, and 12+ reps for endurance. Refer to the total rep range in Prilepin's chart to organize your entire session and you'll be prepared with a solid foundation. Above all, focus on proper technique and a gradual progression to prevent injury. Remember—injured athletes can't play, no matter how good they are.

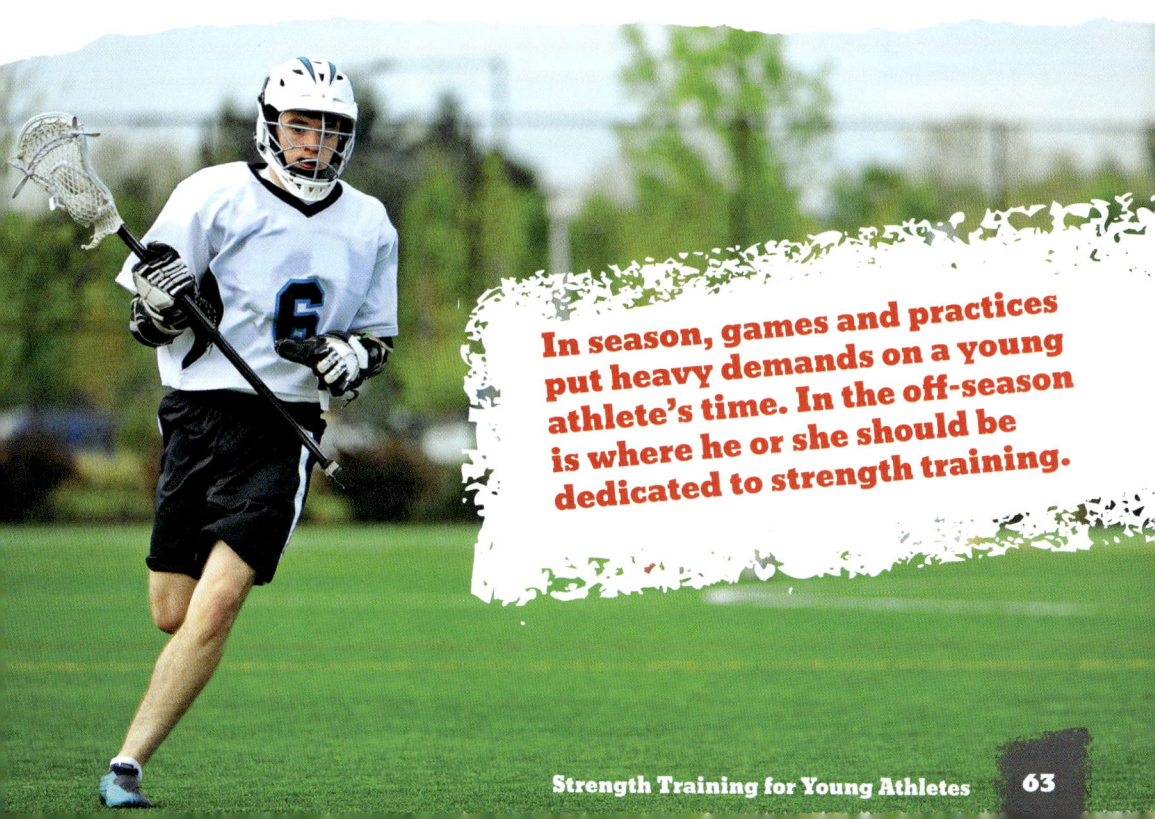

In season, games and practices put heavy demands on a young athlete's time. In the off-season is where he or she should be dedicated to strength training.

CONSIDERATIONS FOR A COMPETITIVE SEASON

Competitive athletes tend to cycle through phases throughout the year. Your sport's off-season, pre-season, in-season, and post-season place different demands upon the body. Therefore, you want to utilize these periods to your advantage and balance them with your strength training.

The off-season is your chance to build and truly develop physically, as you're not pulled away to practices and games. As you have more time and energy, you can dedicate it to strength training. Aim for 2–4 workouts per week during the off-season, depending on experience level and comfort. These workouts can be relatively intense in comparison to other phases, as you'll have time to recover.

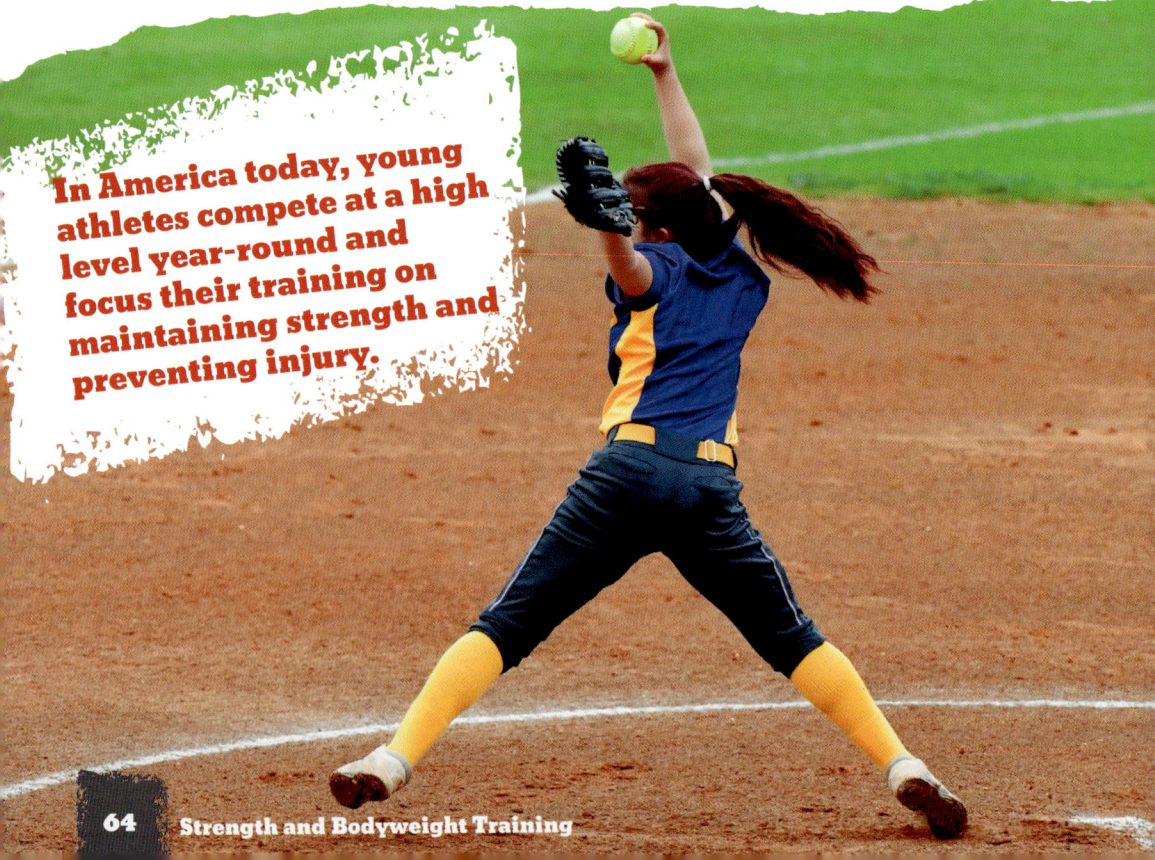

In America today, young athletes compete at a high level year-round and focus their training on maintaining strength and preventing injury.

As pre-season approaches, you'll want to reduce the amount of time in the gym to start preparing specifically for playing your sport. Typically, 2–3 sessions of high intensity, but short duration are appropriate. Once you're in-season, the focus of strength training shifts to maintenance. Usually, 1–3 sessions per week geared to balance out the training demands and maintain function should suffice. Finally, as the post-season approaches, use strength training to peak. Strength training during the post-season should be short sets and reps of moderate to high intensity—such as a few moderately heavy squats or powerful rows.

While this is the pattern of elite athletes, it's not often the case for young athletes. Today, more and more athletes train and compete at a high level year-round, whether in one or multiple sports. If this is your case, train as if you were in-season always. Injury prevention and maintenance are of utmost priority. Work with a certified strength coach to develop a plan that will keep you healthy and performing at your peak.

TEXT-DEPENDENT QUESTIONS

1. In which portion of your competitive season would you want to train for maximum muscle size? Why?
2. What are the six load vectors of sports?
3. Define peak height velocity, and explain its role in youth strength training.

RESEARCH PROJECT

Who is the youngest American Olympic weightlifter to compete in a world championship? Research information on this individual and put together a short essay on his or her history of getting into the sport.

WORDS TO UNDERSTAND

agonist/antagonist—muscles that produce force in opposite directions; the agonist muscle does the concentric action while the antagonist works concentrically to control or prevent it

epiphyseal plates—cartilaginous plates at the end of long bones that allow for growth

thoracic—of, relating to, located within, or involving the part of the body between the neck and the abdomen

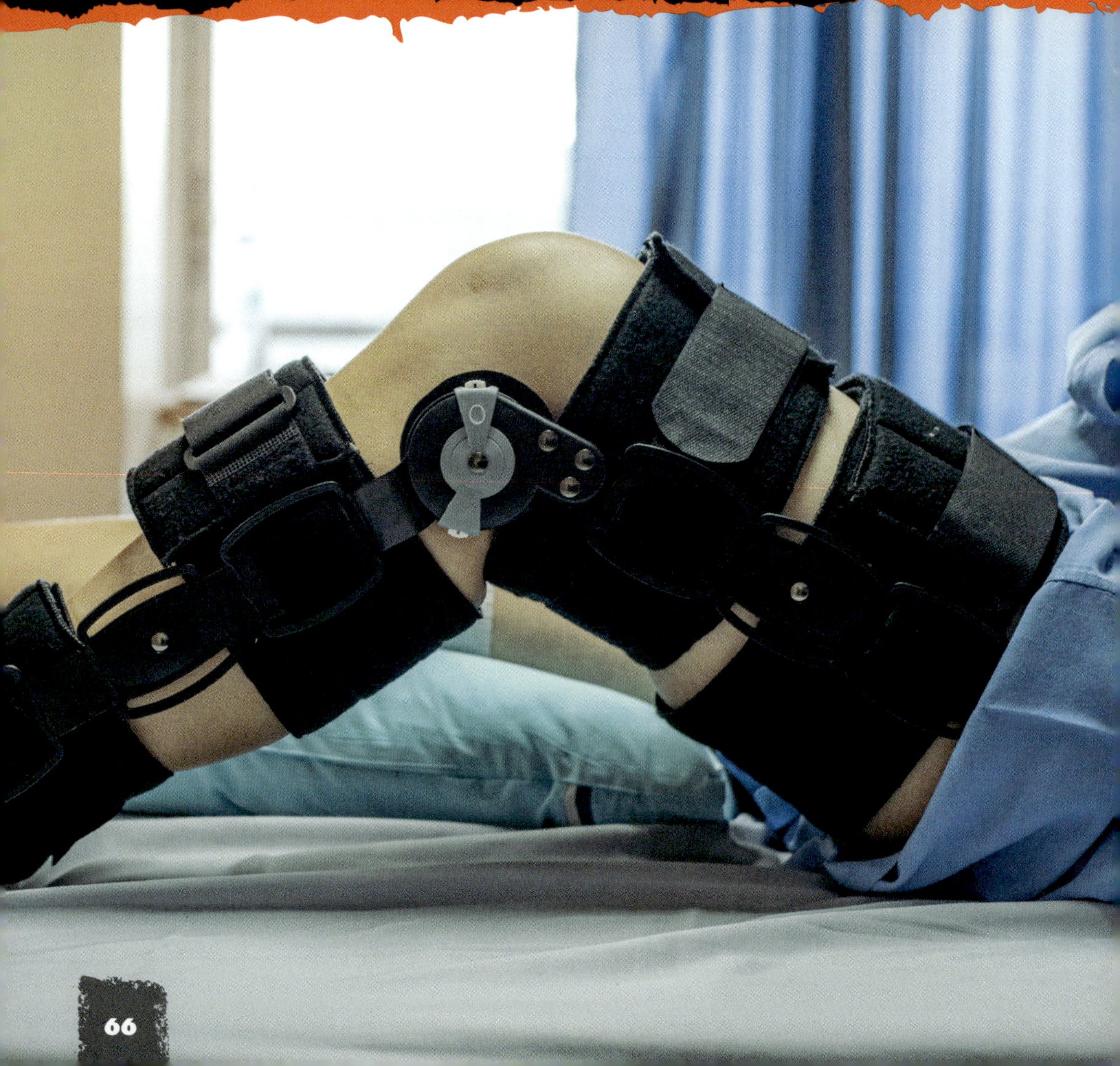

CHAPTER 6
COMMON INJURIES AND HOW TO PREVENT THEM

As with all activities, strength training comes with some injury risk. However, we can mitigate that with proper instruction, management, and strength progression. According to the *Journal of Strength and Conditioning Research*, trunk injuries are the most common weightlifting injuries that send people between ages 14 and 30 to the emergency room. Other common injuries associated with lifting include:

> Muscle strains or tears
> Herniated discs
> Bone fractures
> Growth plate issues

MUSCLE STRAIN OR TEARS

Muscle strains, also known as pulled muscles, result from an overstretching of the tissue. In strength training, these are most common in the lower back, shoulders, neck, hamstrings, or quadriceps. They tend to come in three grades. A Grade I strain only means a few fibers are torn, and, while painful, normal function remains. Grade II causes mild swelling and bruising, as more fibers are damaged. A Grade III strain, or tear, damages the muscle all the way through. These are very serious injuries that separate the muscle from its attached tendon, causing incredible pain.

Typically, muscle strains or tears stem from improper training. Maybe your muscles are too fatigued to do what's required. Or maybe you miss an adequate warm-up, and your muscles are too cold to stretch that far and fast. In order to prevent a muscle strain, always warm-up and develop enough strength to match the demands of your session. Never attempt a maximal effort lift without proper biomechanics, requisite core strength, a spotter, and multiple warm-up sets.

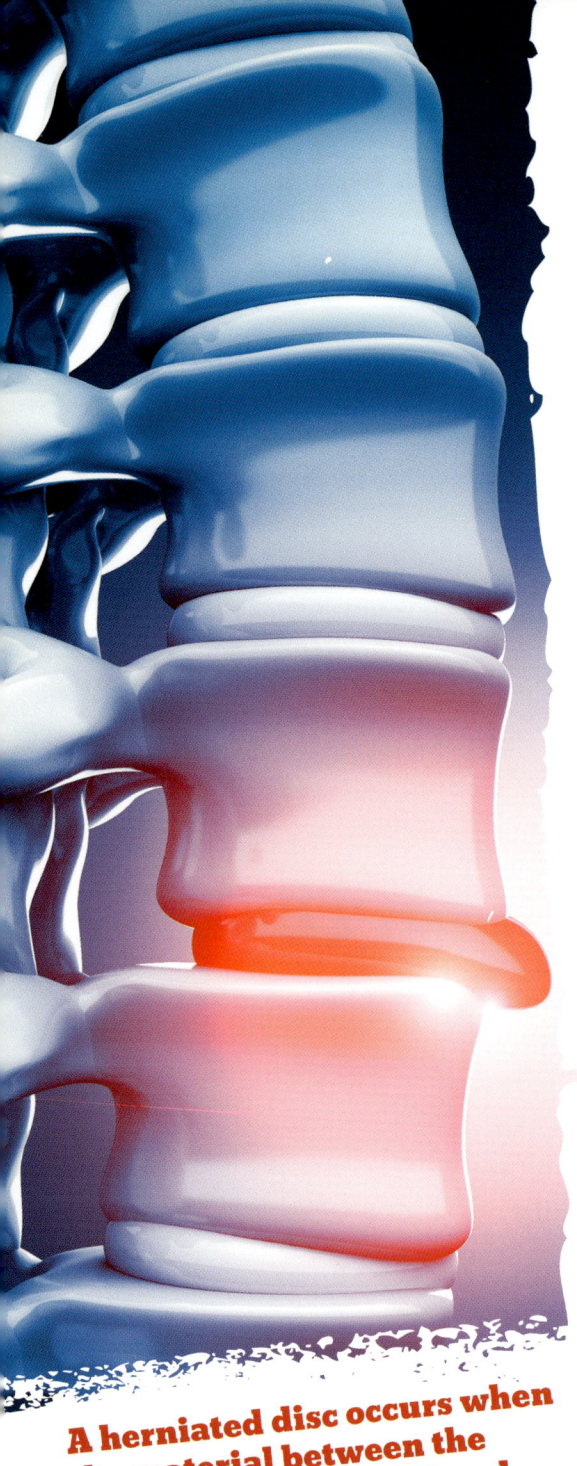

HERNIATED DISCS

Your spinal column contains a series of several vertebrae stacked atop each other. In between each bone lies a layer of cushion known as a disc. Made of collagen fibers, these discs form the shape of a jelly donut. In absence of injury, these little donuts act as the perfect pillows to absorb shock. Sometimes, however, injury, strain, or old age can cause slippage, forcing the inside jelly out of the donut. Due to this displacement, the disc bulges out and presses on nearby nerves.

Herniated discs usually start as mild low back pain, and they progress as pressure increases. Prevent disc injuries by properly loading the spine and bracing the core throughout all strength training exercises.

BONE FRACTURES

Fractures from weightlifting are rarely the result of exercise itself. Rather, bone fractures occur mostly from unsafe lifting conditions. For example, someone could fall off

A herniated disc occurs when the material between the vertebrae is displaced and presses against the spinal cord.

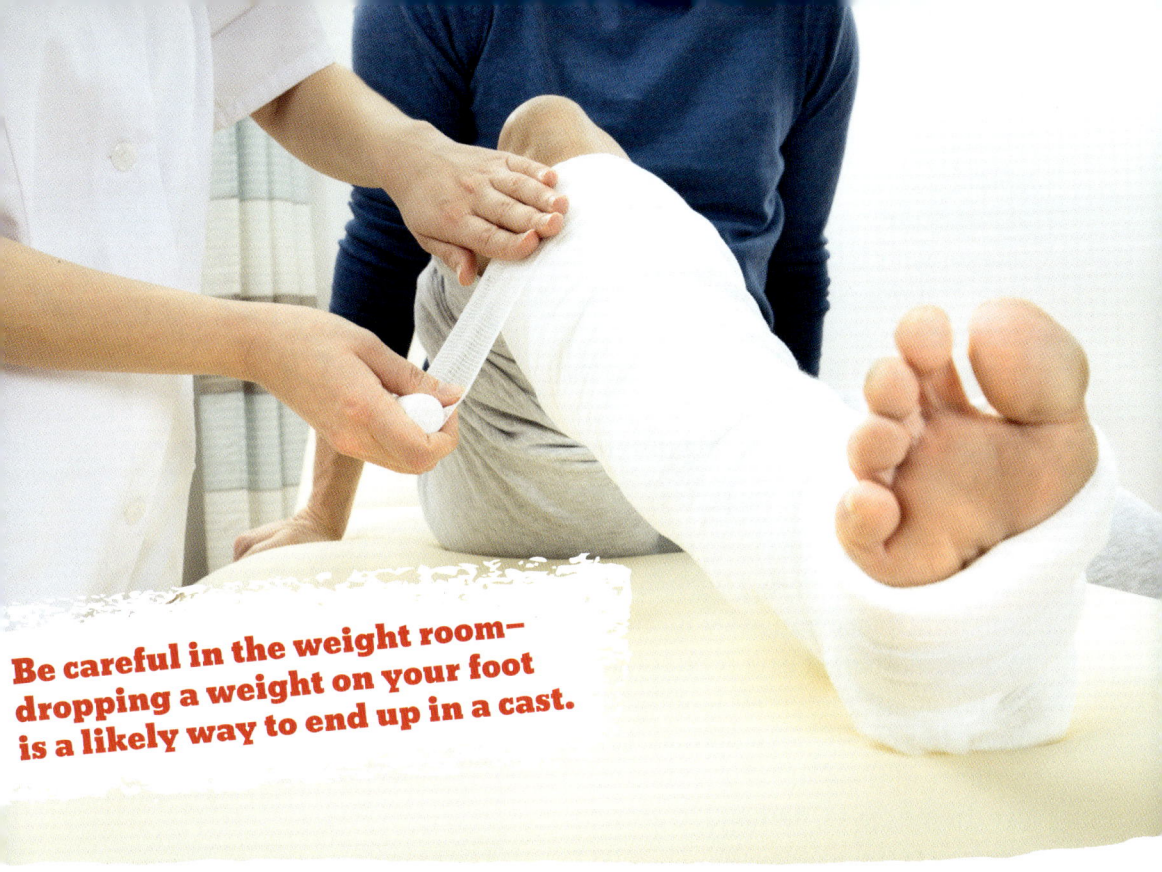

Be careful in the weight room—dropping a weight on your foot is a likely way to end up in a cast.

a pull-up bar and break his or her arm or drop a heavy weight on his or her foot and fracture a toe. To avoid fractures, always lift with a spotter, remove any obstacles, and take care when picking up and putting down weights.

GROWTH PLATE ISSUES

Growth plates, or **epiphyseal plates**, consist of cartilage and sit at the end of new bones. They essentially provide a soft, stretchy gap for our bones to grow into as they expand. Thanks to growth plates, we're able to get taller than we were as infants. Once we reach full maturation, however, these growth plates close and harden into full ossified material.

You may have heard that strength training will harm your growth plates, stunting your growth. That is categorically false. Several reputable organizations, such as the American Orthopaedic Society for Sports Medicine and the American Academy of Pediatrics, agree that a well-structured strength training program is safe.

The problem, again, lies in going too hard too soon. Refering back to the SAID principle, if you ask your body to do something it isn't prepared for, it'll adapt somehow. In growing teens, this could mean damaging the cartilage at the ends of your bones. In extreme cases, damage to growth plates is certainly possible. However, it's easily avoidable. Instead of worrying about an injury, start light and work your way up.

HOW TO AVOID INJURY

Typically, the aforementioned injuries stem from loading too heavily, too quickly. Trying to hit a one-repetition max without proper preparation is a surefire way to get hurt, but don't blame the heavy weights. Researchers have shown that young athletes are exposed to greater forces in sports and

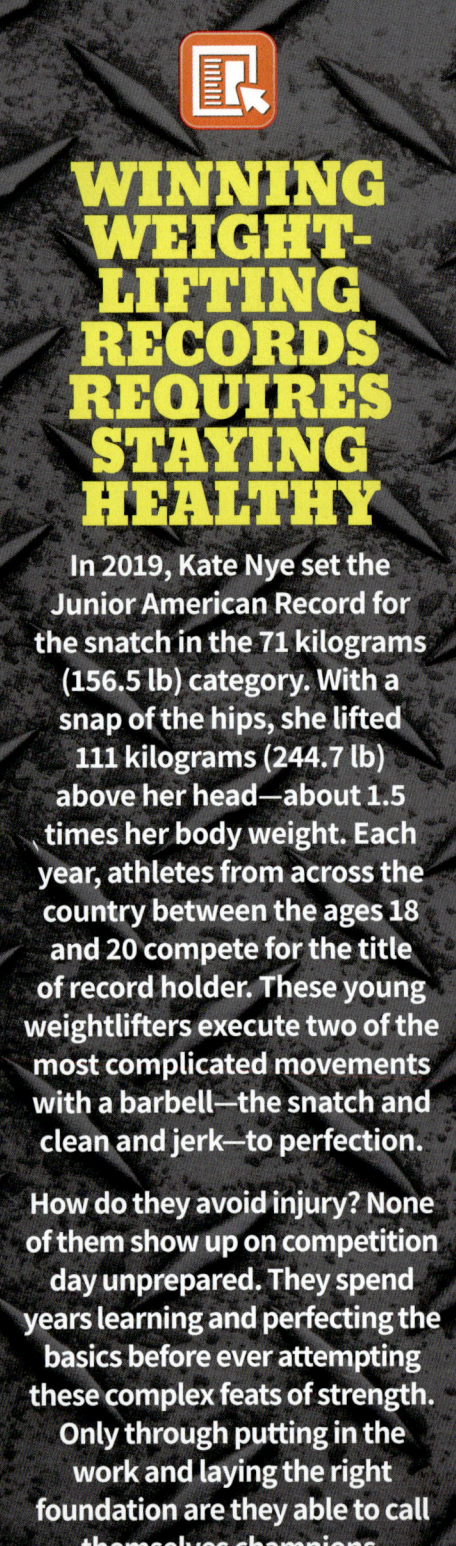

WINNING WEIGHT-LIFTING RECORDS REQUIRES STAYING HEALTHY

In 2019, Kate Nye set the Junior American Record for the snatch in the 71 kilograms (156.5 lb) category. With a snap of the hips, she lifted 111 kilograms (244.7 lb) above her head—about 1.5 times her body weight. Each year, athletes from across the country between the ages 18 and 20 compete for the title of record holder. These young weightlifters execute two of the most complicated movements with a barbell—the snatch and clean and jerk—to perfection.

How do they avoid injury? None of them show up on competition day unprepared. They spend years learning and perfecting the basics before ever attempting these complex feats of strength. Only through putting in the work and laying the right foundation are they able to call themselves champions.

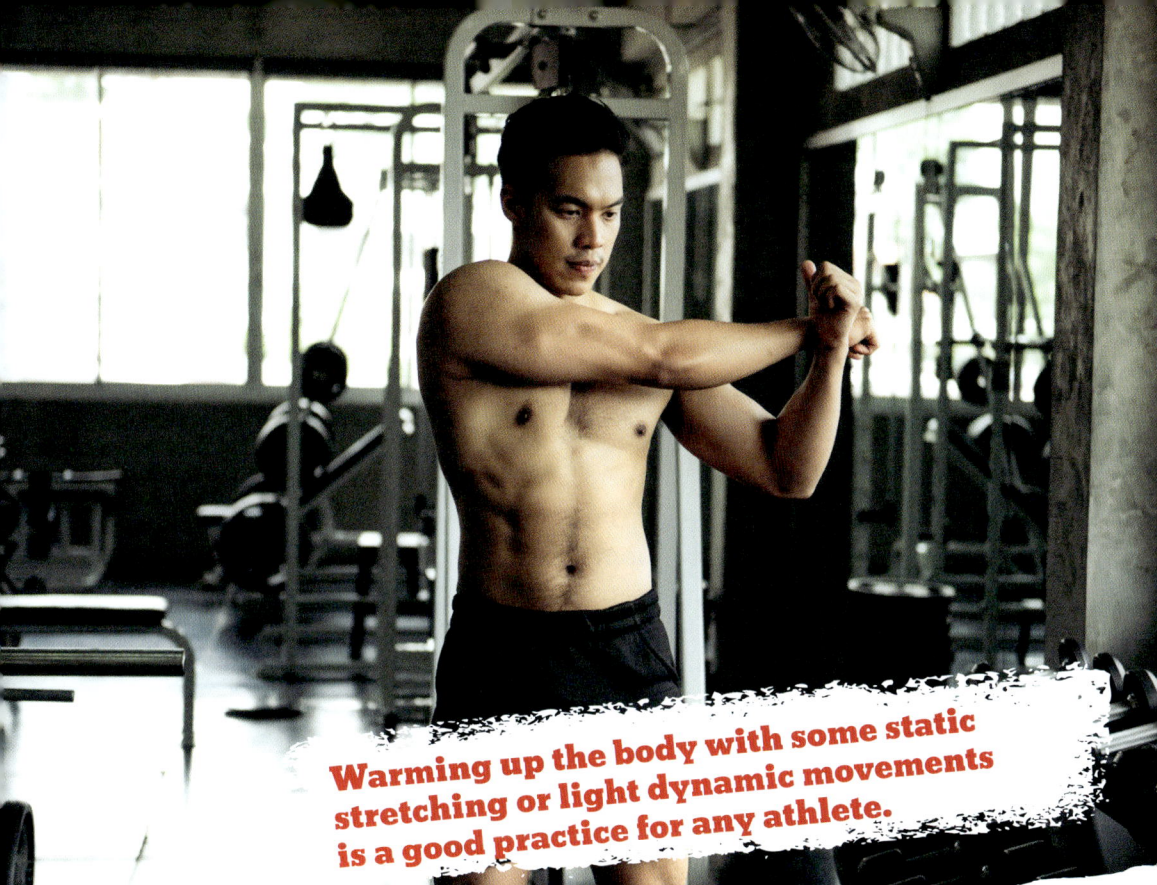

Warming up the body with some static stretching or light dynamic movements is a good practice for any athlete.

recreational activities than maximal strength tests. It's just that they're prepared for these events through practice, a good warm-up, and progression.

Warm-Up and Mobility

A good warm-up requires much more than static stretching. Rather, it's a progressive, structured activation period designed to prepare you for the upcoming activity. Injury prevention depends on this fact, as the ill-prepared are more likely to get hurt.

Your strength training warm-up should always start with its namesake—getting warm. Light aerobic activity elevates circulation and stimulates alertness. Moreover, it helps muscles, tendons, and connective tissue become more elastic, allowing you to get into deeper ranges of motion. Following 2–5 minutes of heart rate elevation, include a period of mobilization specific to your lift.

For example, if your lift calls for squats, bench press, and pull-ups, you'll want to target the hips, ankles, shoulders, and upper back. Activities such as dynamic hip flexor stretches, hip circles, leg swings, and calf stretches open up your lower body, while cat/cow, arm circles, and child's pose work your upper body.

For more information about these exercises, consult the ACE Exercise Library under the Internet Resources section at the end of this book.

Core Activation and Training

A large portion of injury stems from a weak core. Your core represents the connection between your upper and lower body, and it acts as the solid base through which you transfer force. More than just a six-pack, your core forms a cylinder between your diaphragm and pelvic floor muscles, wrapping all the way around the body. Some experts include the glutes and lats in core training as well since they control pelvic and **thoracic** positioning.

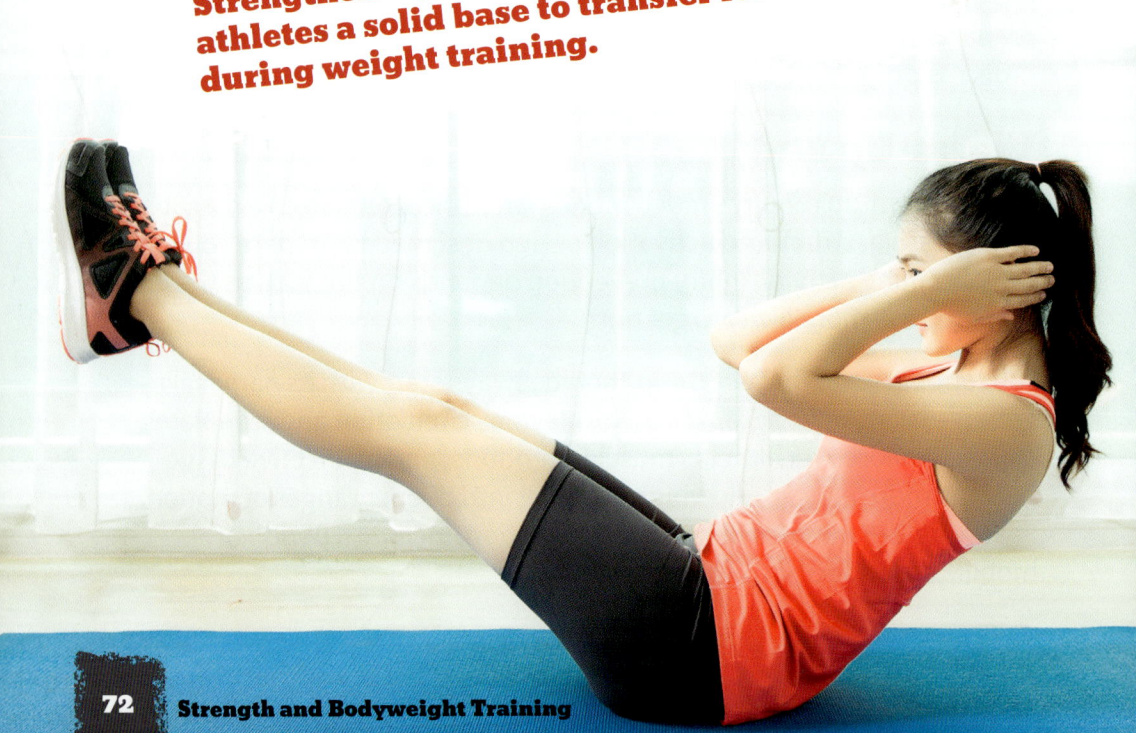

Strengthening the core will give athletes a solid base to transfer force during weight training.

Think of your core as the pillar between the floor and the ceiling of buildings. When solid, the building stays safe. If this base is compromised, however, something has to give. Learning to build and brace your core causes a similar effect. You want to be able to withstand difficult loads and fight any unexpected instability. Therefore, you have to train your core to remain active throughout movement. While your arms are doing one thing and your legs are doing another, your core should remain solid as a rock.

Train your core stability by incorporating plank variations, dead bugs, bird dogs, glute bridges, and other stabilization exercises into your warm-up. These exercises serve as a reminder to your neuromuscular system just before lifting. That way, when it's time to lift weights, your core is ready to go.

Regular Strength Training

Oddly enough, regular strength training can actually help prevent weight training-related injuries. It's just like anything else—the more you practice something, the better you get at it. To a point, strength training follows the same rule. You'll be more comfortable in the movements, you'll get stronger, and you'll be more injury-resistant.

That is, assuming you maintain a healthy balance. If you only bench press, your other muscles will get left behind. As these "mirror muscles" grow, their strength overpowers their counterparts, and your joints creep into bad positions. All **agonists**—or muscles that are applying force—have a corresponding **antagonist**—the muscles that provide opposition. To avoid injury, train both equally, as well as any secondary stabilizing muscles.

At its core, injury occurs because your muscles weren't strong enough to withstand the forces applied. This can happen over time, in the case of muscular imbalance and overuse, or it can happen in an instant, such as a muscle tear. A well-balanced strength training program helps your muscles respond to dangerous situations. By training the body over and over again to withstand the external demands of a sport (aka lifting), you prevent injury.

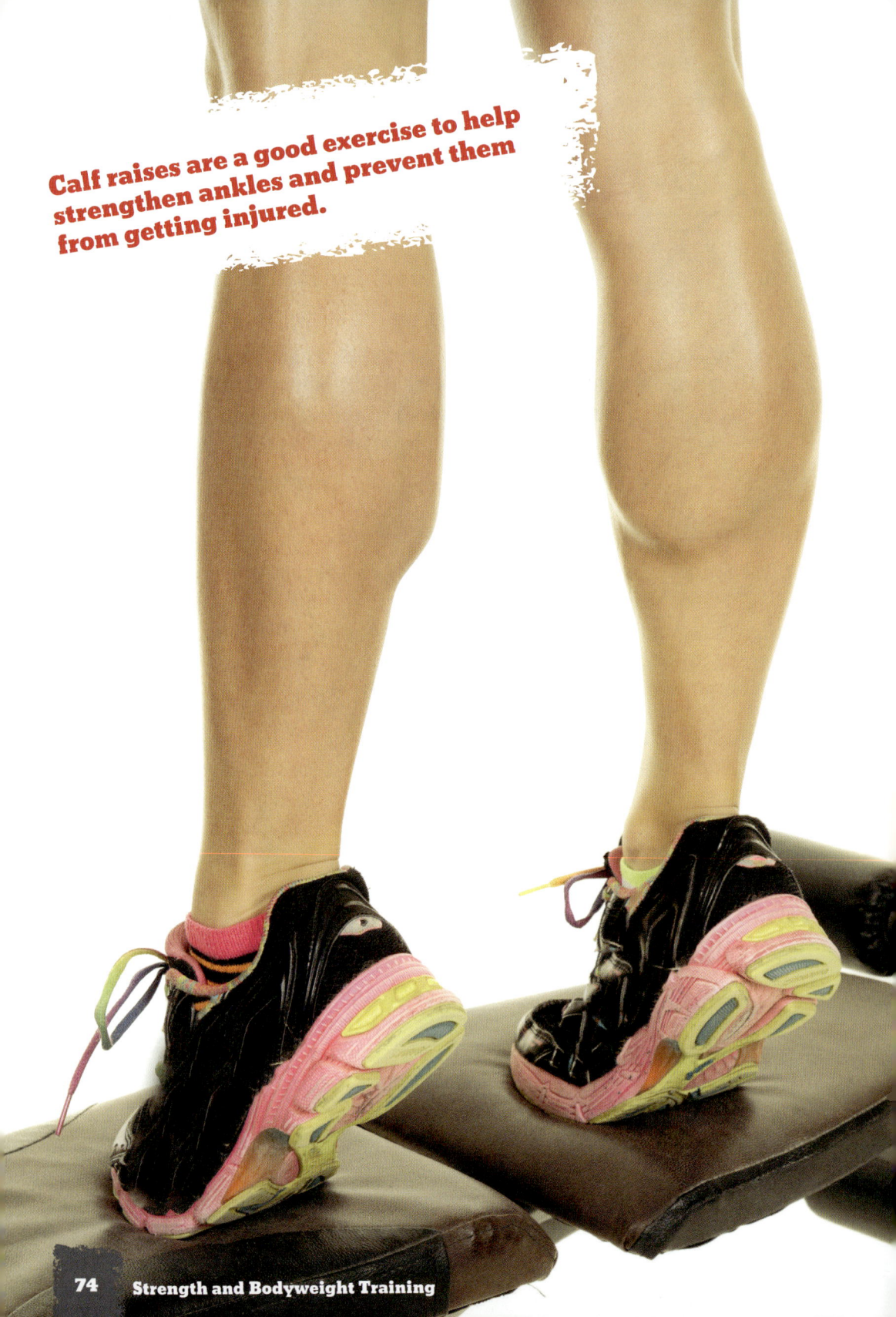

Calf raises are a good exercise to help strengthen ankles and prevent them from getting injured.

 Check out these examples of ankle-strengthening prehab exercises.

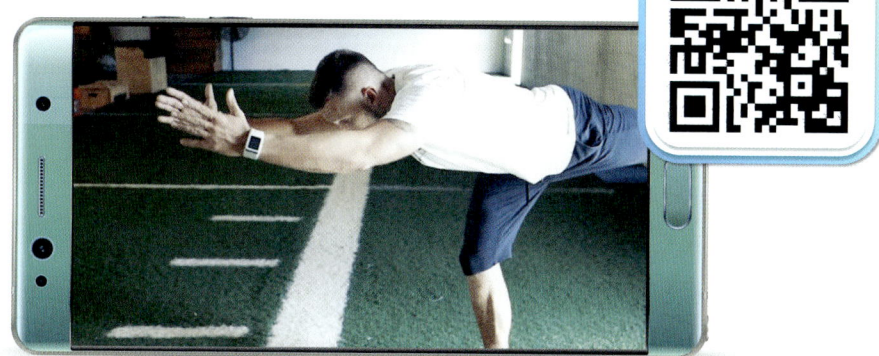

Sport-Specific Prehab

If you're an athlete, pay attention. Injury risks are often greater in sports than they are in the gym. Prehab is short for "pre-rehabilitation," which essentially means stopping injury before it occurs. While no one can

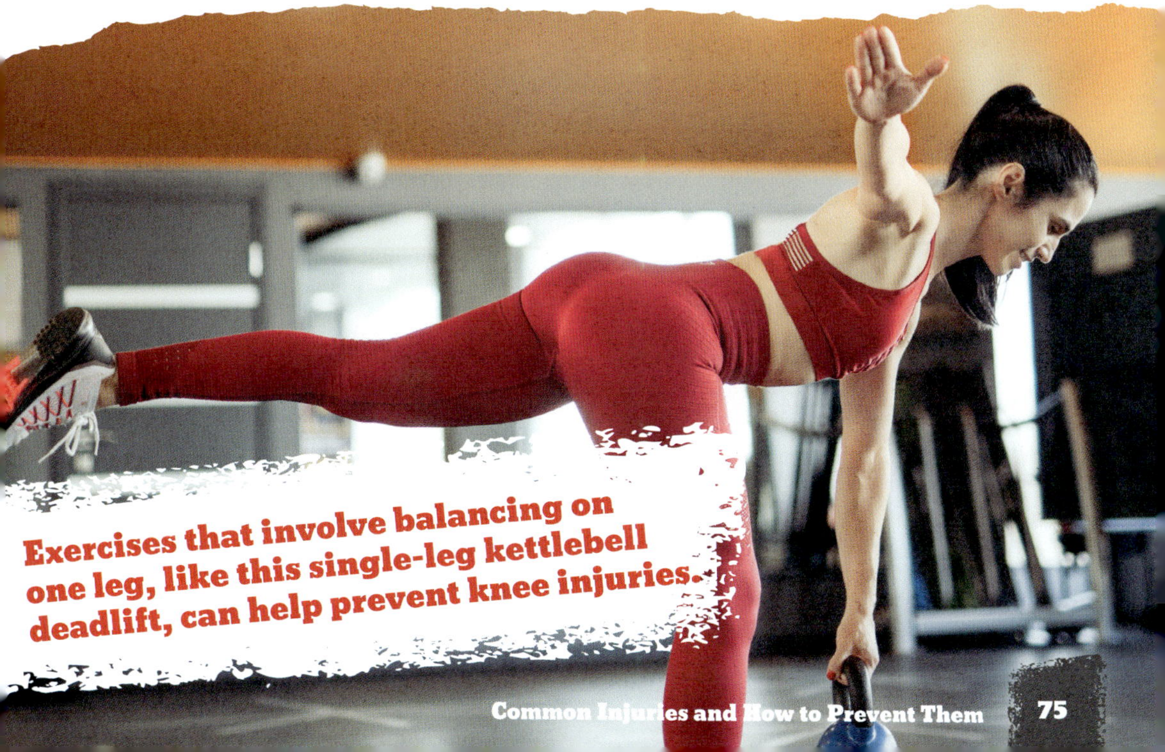

Exercises that involve balancing on one leg, like this single-leg kettlebell deadlift, can help prevent knee injuries.

see the future (and completely avoiding ALL injury is impossible), the following exercises can help keep your joints healthy.

Exercises to prevent ankle injuries:

> Calf raises and stretching
> Banded inversion/eversion
> Banded plantar and dorsiflexion
> Balancing on unstable surfaces

Exercises to prevent knee injuries:

> Clamshells
> Single-leg balance
> Mini band walks
> Nordic hamstring curls
> Single-leg RDL, squat, and lunge variations

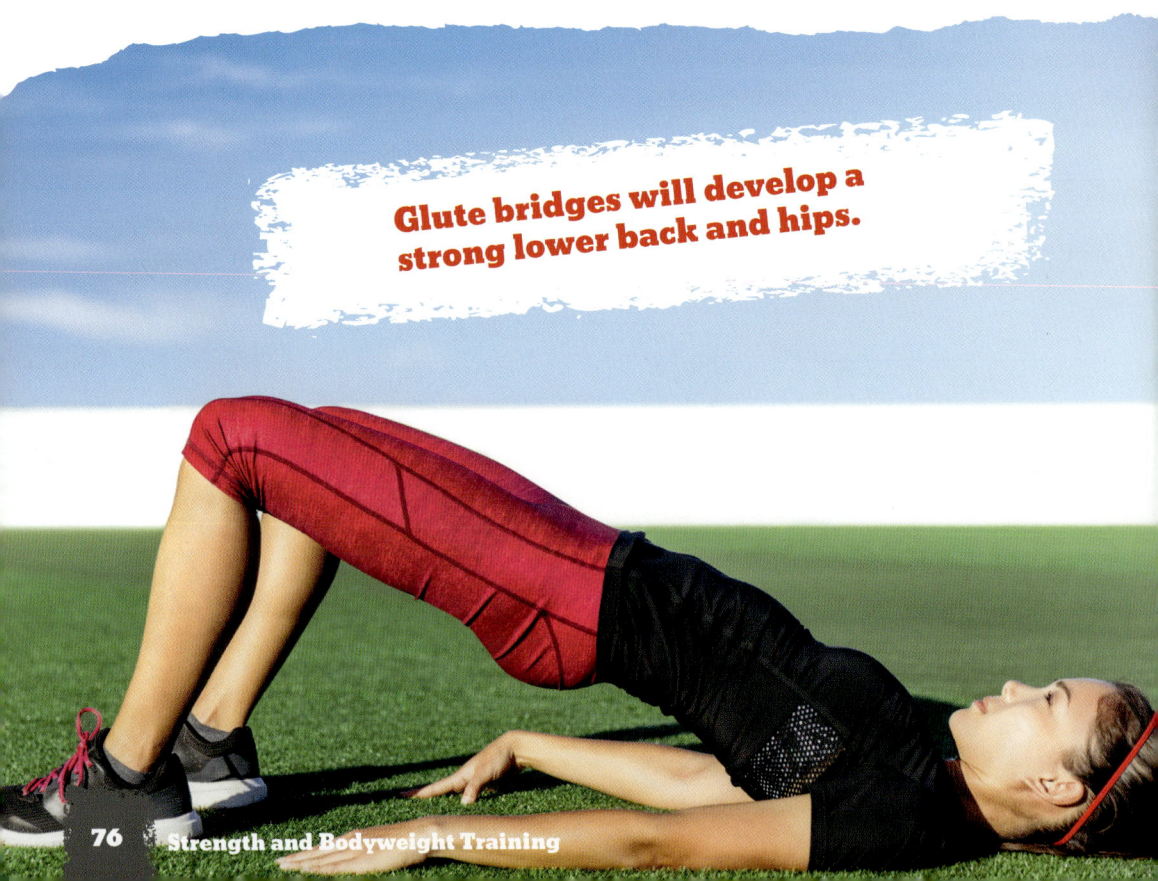

Glute bridges will develop a strong lower back and hips.

Exercises to prevent hip/low back injuries:

> Pelvic tilts
> Dead bugs
> Anti-rotation exercises (Pallof press, ½ kneel presses, etc.)
> Plank variations
> Glute bridges

Exercises to prevent elbow/shoulder injuries:

> Y, T, W raises
> Banded internal/external rotation
> Scapular push-ups
> Row variations
> Kettlebell holds

For more information about these exercises, consult the ACE Exercise Library under the Internet Resources section at the end of this book.

TEXT-DEPENDENT QUESTIONS

1. What exercises or movements would be appropriate as part of a warm-up for barbell squats?

2. What is an epiphyseal plate? Highlight its place in strength training and how to avoid injuring it.

3. What role does the core play in injury prevention?

RESEARCH PROJECT

Using the ACE Exercise Library referenced in the Internet Resources section, look up 2–3 exercises that help prevent injury at each joint. Then choose one of the most common strength training injuries (muscle strains or tears, herniated discs, bone fractures, or growth plate issues) and design a practical prehab program for it.

WORDS TO UNDERSTAND

anterior chain—a collection of muscles that work in tandem to control the front half of the body, such as the pectoralis major, quadriceps, and iliopsoas

regress—to move backward; go back

scapulohumeral rhythm—the degree of movement at the scapula in comparison to the humerus, which is roughly 1:2 during passive motion

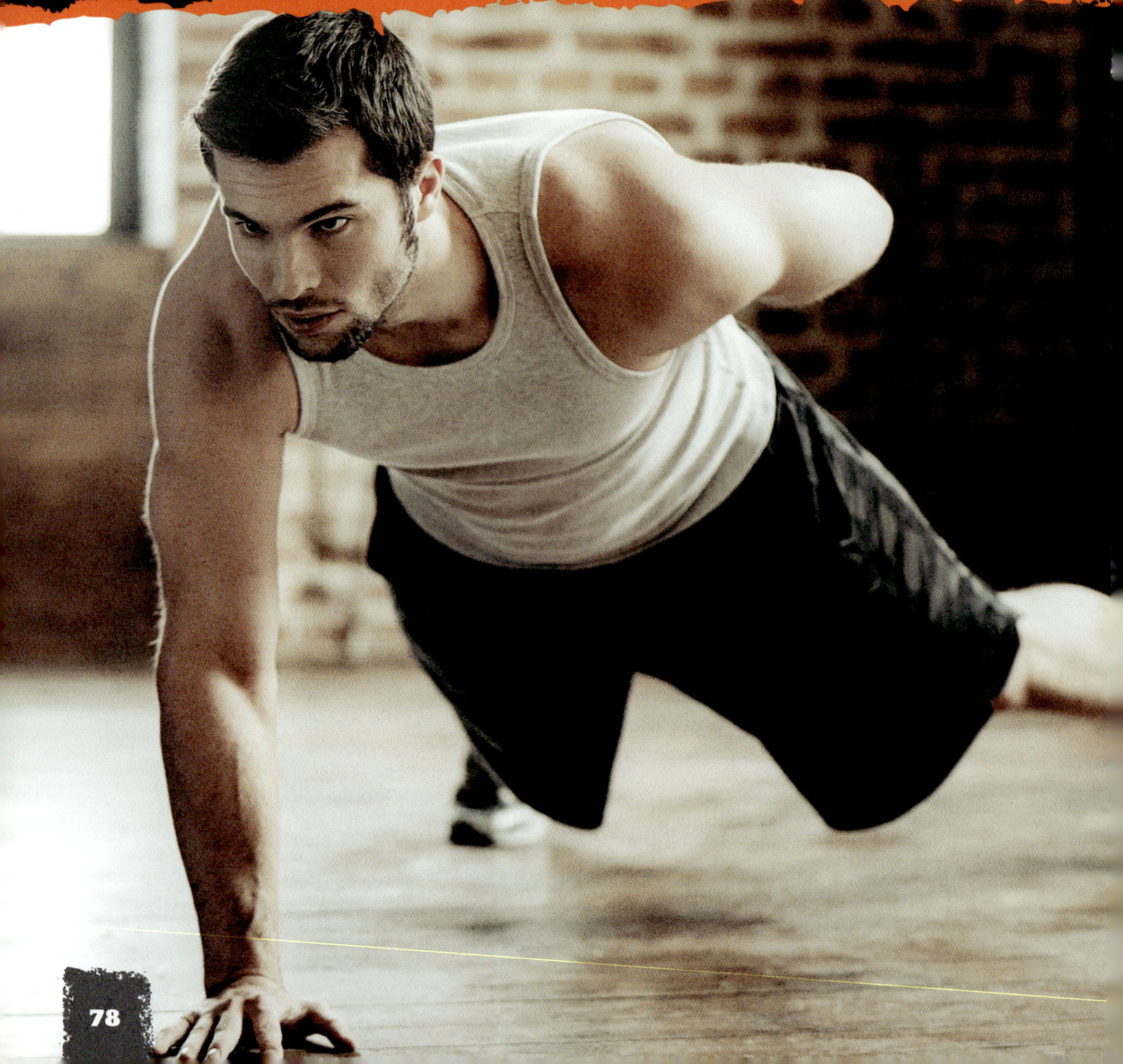

CHAPTER 7
STRENGTH TRAINING EXERCISES

If you've read this far, you're probably wondering, "What exactly do I do in the gym? And how?"

To help you get started, we're going to go through some of the top exercises in each loading pattern. Pick at least one movement from each of the categories below, follow the sets and reps from above, and get to work!

UPPER BODY PUSH

The awareness of postural positioning is critical in weightlifting. In upper body mechanics, your arm and shoulder are designed to move together in something known as **scapulohumeral rhythm.** This natural biomechanical factor dictates that for every degree of passive elevation in the humerus (upper arm bone), the scapula (shoulder blade) will upwardly rotate by half a degree. This means the arm raises at twice the rate of your shoulder blade. This changes slightly as load is added, but a drastic change can disrupt natural function. Tight, weak, or otherwise inactive muscles around the shoulder blade is a common weightlifting issue, increasing injury risk. Push-ups affix your arms to the floor, helping train those smaller muscles as you press up.

PUSH-UP

As noted previously, if you can learn how to do push-ups properly with your body weight, you'll set an ideal foundation for all types of pressing. Some people struggle at the start, and that's perfectly normal. Modifications of the push-up, such as push-ups from the knees or pressing against an elevated bar, decrease the difficulty. Choose whatever variation you can do with pristine form until you get strong enough to progress.

To execute a perfect push-up, do the following:

1. Start in a high plank position with wrists underneath your shoulders so that your forearms are perpendicular to the floor. Hands can lie slightly outside of the shoulders.//
2. Keep the spine neutral and engage the core before beginning the movement. A regular push-up begins on the floor with your legs extended and weight resting on the toes and palms. If this position is too advanced, either drop to the knees or elevate the hands.
3. From the start position, try to pull the floor apart with your hands. This will help set your shoulders in place before you descend.
4. Maintain this position as you slowly lower the torso down to just above the floor. Drive the elbows back behind you and avoid flaring them outward.
5. Pause briefly at the bottom and press back up to the start position. Avoid arching the back or sticking your glutes in the air as you complete the rep. If this seems impossible, try a modification.
6. Repeat as needed until all reps are complete.

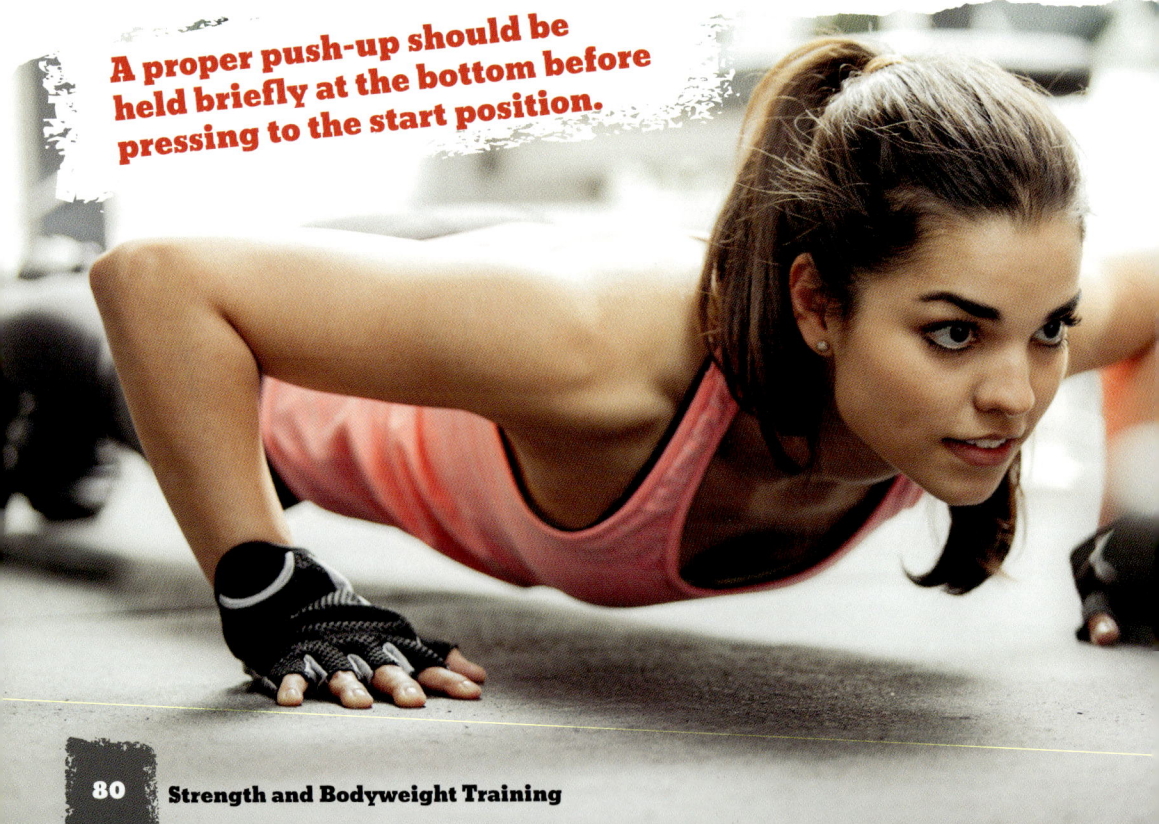

A proper push-up should be held briefly at the bottom before pressing to the start position.

If you can't complete the rep without arching the lower back, elevating the chest, or raising your glutes in the air, **regress** to a less difficult modification until strength is further developed.

BARBELL BENCH

A barbell bench press mimics an upside down push-up. Since you'll press the weight directly above your chest, always start with an empty barbell and work with a spotter to avoid injury.

1. Lie face-up on the bench with feet touching the floor. Your tailbone, mid-back, and head should all be resting on the bench.
2. Position yourself underneath the bar so that it's directly above your eyes. Grip the bar with the same hand position as a push-up, wrists just outside the shoulders.
3. Using a spotter to help you, press up slightly to unrack the bar. Bring it just above the chest so your arms are perpendicular to the floor. Pull your shoulder blades together as if you were trying to break the barbell in half (don't worry, you won't).
4. Just like a reverse push up, pull the bar slowly to the chest. Keep your elbows down rather than pointing out and away from you.
5. Pause briefly once the bar touches the sternum. Squeeze the glutes as you press the weight back up. Make sure not to let your head, glutes, or other parts of your body leave the bench as you press.
6. Complete the rep when your arms are locked out and repeat as necessary.

OTHER UPPER BODY PUSHING OPTIONS

As you continue through your strength training regimen, you may want to explore the following other upper body pushing exercises.

> Other push-up variations
> Dumbbell bench press
> Overhead press

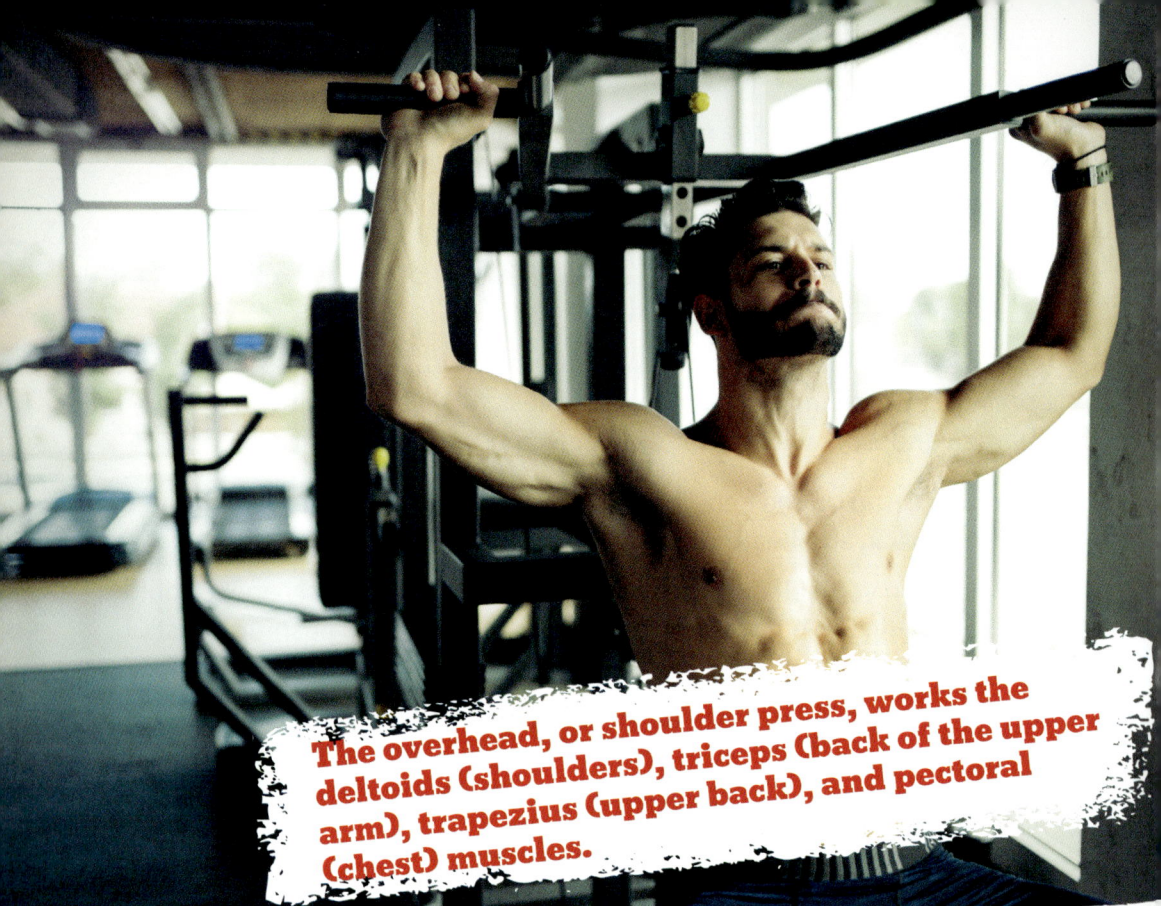

The overhead, or shoulder press, works the deltoids (shoulders), triceps (back of the upper arm), trapezius (upper back), and pectoral (chest) muscles.

> Incline press
> Push Press
> Any single-arm variation of the above

UPPER BODY PULL

Similar to upper body pushing, it's smart to start pulling exercises with bodyweight- and groove-efficient biomechanical patterns. One of the best places to start is the inverted row, where you're pulling your body up to a bar.

Inverted Row

If you have access to suspension cables such as TRX, set them up at an appropriate length for comfortable, full-range pulling. Otherwise, set up a barbell in the rack near chest height. Before beginning, grip the implement and walk your feet forward so you're leaning back. The closer you are to parallel with the ground, the more difficult the row. When ready to begin, proceed as follows:

1. Grab the implement with two hands just outside of the shoulders. Start with either an overhand position (palms facing the ground) or a neutral position (palms facing each other).
2. Keeping your core engaged, walk your feet forward while leaning back, until you reach a comfortable angle with arms outstretched. Your body should look like a straight line, head to toe.
3. With your shoulders away from your ears, squeeze your shoulder blades together as you punch your elbows behind you. Continue pulling until the elbows clear your body.

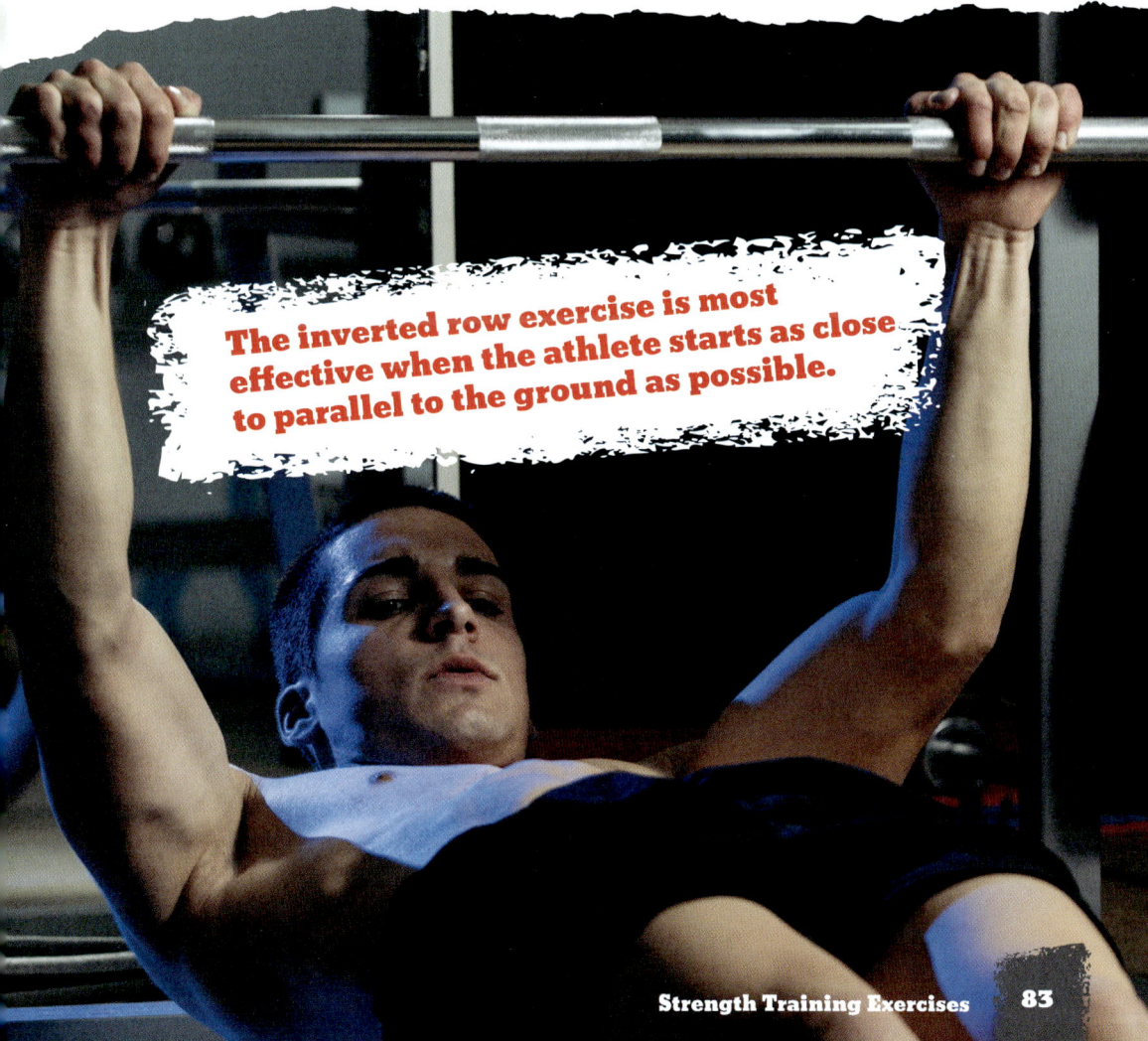

The inverted row exercise is most effective when the athlete starts as close to parallel to the ground as possible.

4. Squeeze lightly at the top and then slowly lower the body back to the starting position.
5. Repeat as needed.

Pull-Ups/Chin-Ups

Pull-ups are a progression above the inverted row. As your whole body is suspended, you'll need enough strength to lift your entire body weight directly against gravity. If strength is lacking, a resistance band or partner can assist.

1. Grip the bar by wrapping the thumb around it with knuckles flat. Secure your hand in place tightly and hang directly underneath the bar. For pull-ups, have your palms facing away from you. For chin-ups, face your palms toward you.
2. Always start the movement by sliding your scapulae down before bending at the elbows. Take care to keep the head and spine neutral with the core tight while pulling your chin up over the bar.
3. Slowly lower with the same posture until arms are fully extended.

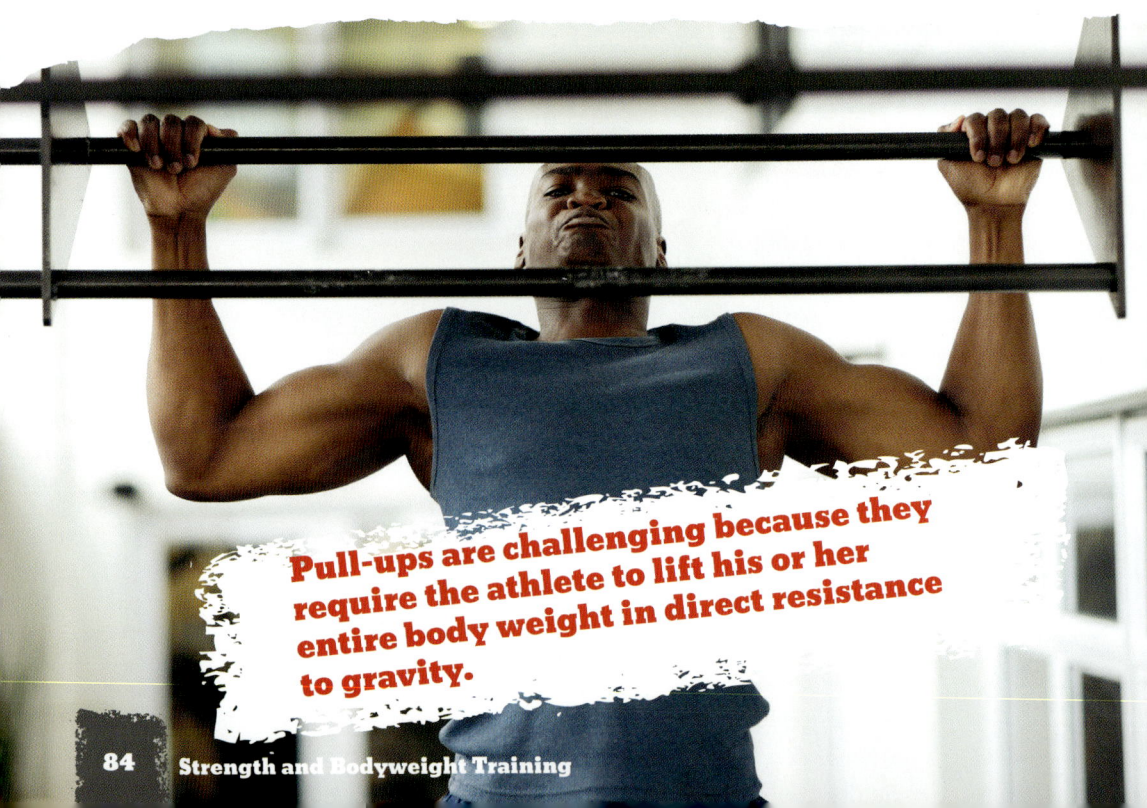

Pull-ups are challenging because they require the athlete to lift his or her entire body weight in direct resistance to gravity.

Other Upper Body Pulling Options:

> Lat pulldown
> Dumbbell bent-over row
> Barbell bent-over row
> Cable row
> Any single-arm variation of the above

LOWER BODY HINGE

Years of sitting in chairs in class or playing video games have made us tight little round balls. Therefore, the hip hinge is one of the most

Experts at the hip hinge can reach the pictured position. Most athletes should stop when a good stretch is felt in the hamstrings.

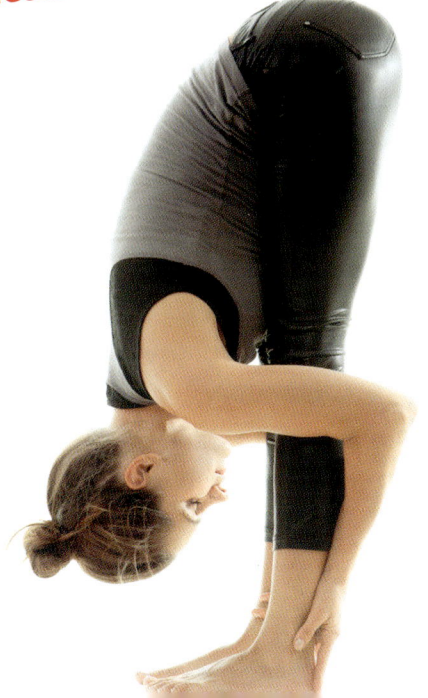

BECOMING THE FITTEST PERSON ON EARTH

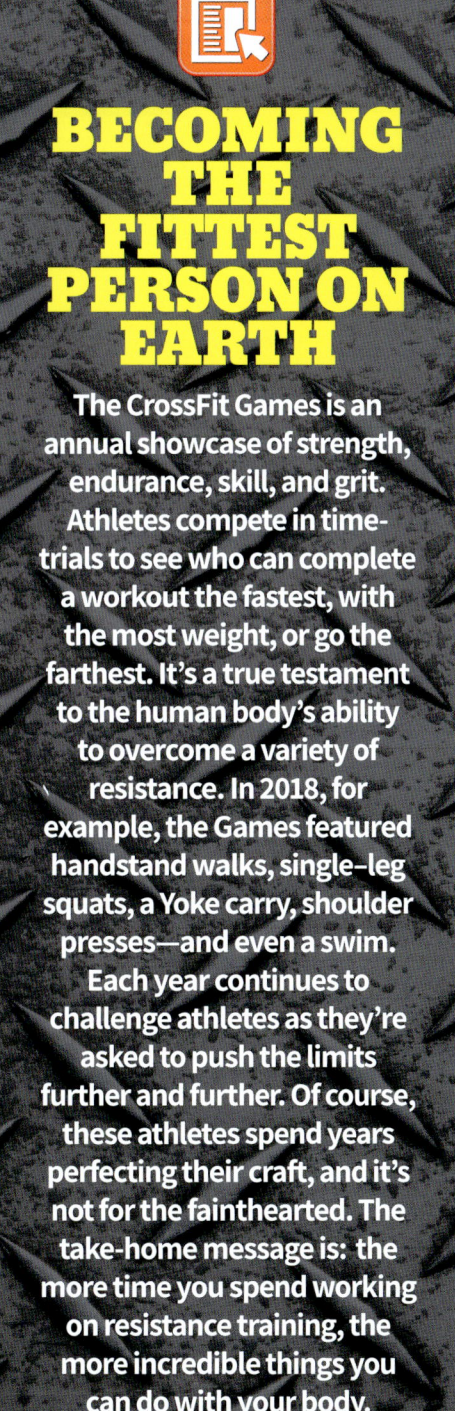

The CrossFit Games is an annual showcase of strength, endurance, skill, and grit. Athletes compete in time-trials to see who can complete a workout the fastest, with the most weight, or go the farthest. It's a true testament to the human body's ability to overcome a variety of resistance. In 2018, for example, the Games featured handstand walks, single–leg squats, a Yoke carry, shoulder presses—and even a swim.

Each year continues to challenge athletes as they're asked to push the limits further and further. Of course, these athletes spend years perfecting their craft, and it's not for the fainthearted. The take-home message is: the more time you spend working on resistance training, the more incredible things you can do with your body.

 **This demonstration video from the Mayo Clinic shows the proper technique for the hip hinge.**

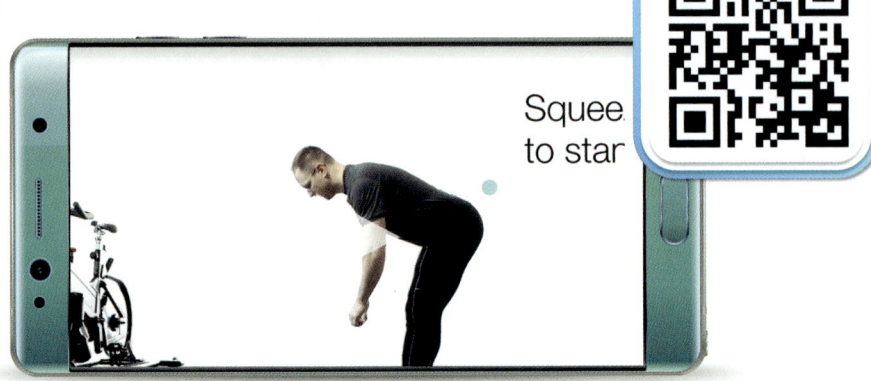

important movements to learn (or re-learn) for a balanced physique. It involves driving your hips backward with a flat back while staying balanced over your midfoot. It's the same position you automatically go into when trying to jump as high as possible, and, coincidentally, being able to hip hinge is key to athletic performance.

Many people fear this exercise, worried that it'll harm their lower back. On the contrary, if you learn to engage the musculature of the hips, hamstrings, and core, you'll build a body resilient against damage.

The Hip Hinge/Romanian Deadlift

1. Begin standing upright with feet hip-width apart. Keeping your core tight and spine neutral, drive your hips behind you, as if you were trying to touch a wall with your glutes.
2. To keep from falling over, lean forward slightly as your torso descends. Think of moving your glutes back and chest forward at the same time.
3. Keep the legs straight, but not locked out as you approach parallel with the ground. Flexibility will limit how far you can go, so hinge until you feel a stretch in your hamstrings. Pause briefly at the bottom.
4. Press your feet into the floor and squeeze your glutes to stand up. Your core should remain engaged during the entire movement, from start to finish.
5. Repeat as necessary.

To progress to weighted Romanian deadlifts, simply hold dumbbells or a barbell in your hands. Keep it tight to your body the entire time, grazing your legs throughout.

One note: avoid craning the neck during the hip hinge. It can be tempting to continue to look upward, but always keep your head neutral. A good cue is holding a PVC pipe or dowel in a straight line down your back with both hands. Throughout the movement, the pipe should keep in contact with the back of your head, mid-back, and hips.

Other Lower Body Hinge Exercises

As you get comfortable with the hip hinge, you can progress to other exercises, such as:

> Glute bridge
> Single-leg glute bridge
> Barbell deadlift
> Trap bar deadlift
> Banded pull-throughs
> Kettlebell swing
> Single-leg RDL (bodyweight or resisted)

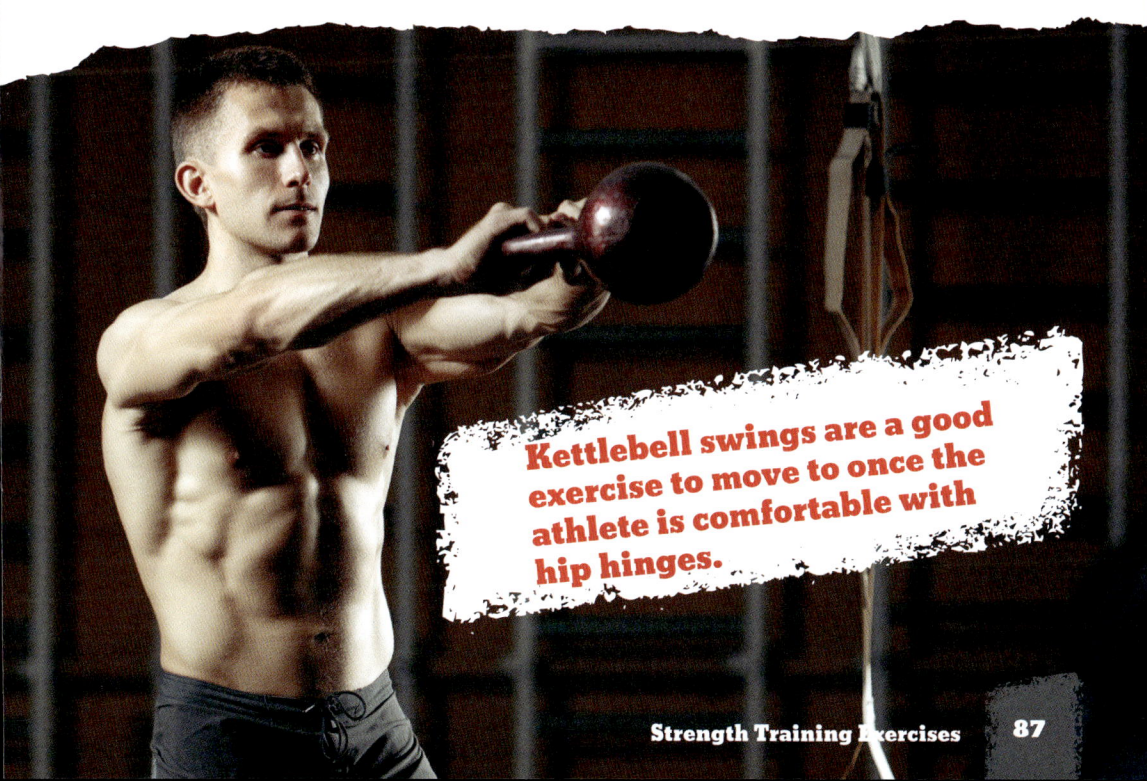

Kettlebell swings are a good exercise to move to once the athlete is comfortable with hip hinges.

LOWER BODY QUAD DOMINANT

Quad dominant movements, while still training the entire legs, place greater emphasis on the **anterior chain**. The squat rules these lower body exercises. Even since we were toddlers, we've been squatting to play with our toys, jump around on the playground, or crawl under fences. Therefore, the squat is a staple in any comprehensive strength training program.

To execute a bodyweight squat:

1. Position the feet just outside the shoulders, toes pointed forward, and arms directly out in front of you for balance.
2. Begin the squat by hinging the hips backward with a flat back and let your torso tilt forward as you descend, heels down and balancing the weight over the center of the foot. It's important to keep your shins vertical and knees behind the toes.

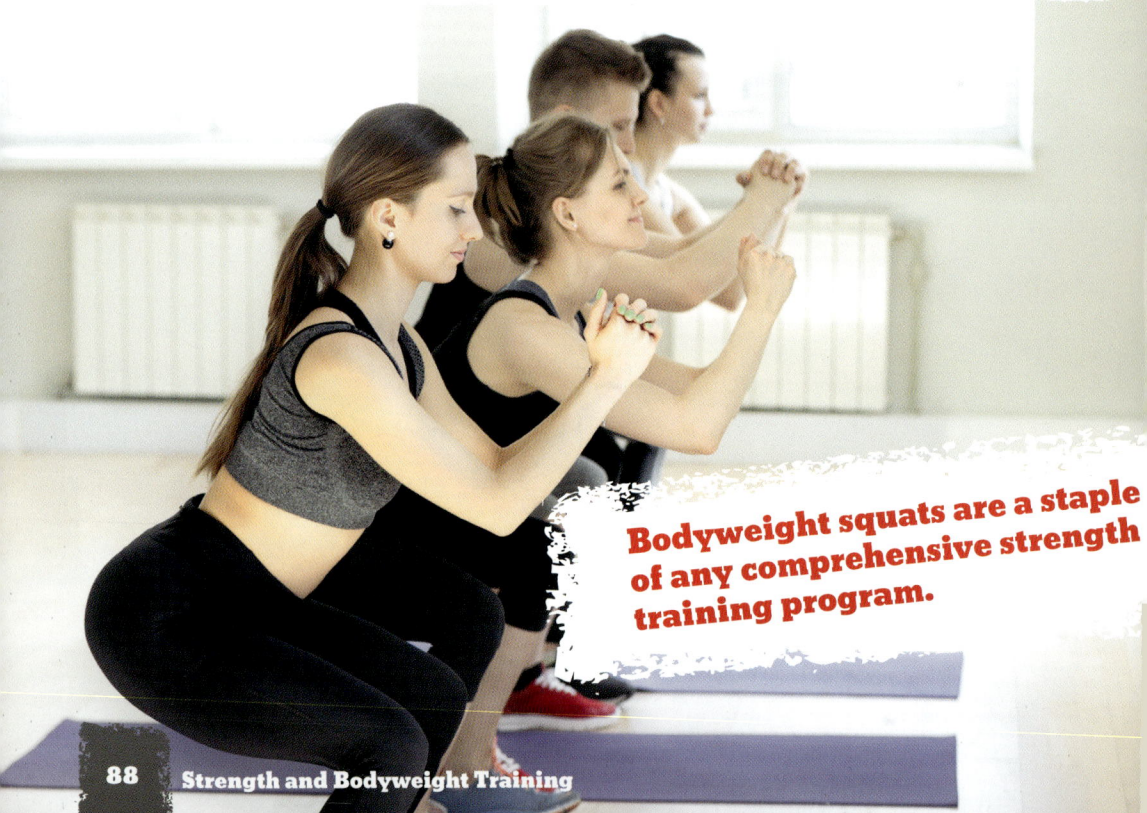

Bodyweight squats are a staple of any comprehensive strength training program.

3. As your hips drop below parallel, keep the knees out, back and core tight. This will help everything stay in line and avoid tucking the tailbone. Reverse the motion to drive yourself back up.

4. Push the knees out and drive your feet into the floor as you extend the hips to come back to standing. Again, take care to keep the shins vertical, upper back tight, and spine neutral.

To add weight, you can progress to a goblet squat. The goblet squat is essentially the same as an air squat while holding a dumbbell, medicine ball, or kettlebell. Adding an anterior load requires much more upper back and core engagement to remain stable. Make sure you can execute the full squat with an upright torso.

Barbell Back Squat

A barbell back squat is slightly more advanced. You'll need a squat rack, a barbell set up at shoulder height, and a partner to spot you before beginning.

To execute a barbell back squat:

1. Stand in the squat rack, reach in front of you, grip the barbell wider than shoulder-width, and pull your body underneath it. Position yourself so the barbell can rest comfortably on the meat of your upper traps, not the neck. Your grip should be comfortable but positioned with wrists straight and elbows stacked underneath the bar.

2. Pressing against the barbell, contract your core, squeeze the glutes, and stand up with the bar on your back. Take a step backward to unrack the bar.

3. Adopt the same stance as a bodyweight squat, brace the spine and core, and descend until legs are parallel with the ground.

4. Drive your feet into the floor, keeping the core engaged and torso upright, to stand up.

Other Lower Body Quad Dominant Exercises

> Front squat
> Overhead squat
> Lunge
> Lateral lunge
> Split squat variation

ROTATIONAL EXERCISES, CARRIES, AND CORE EXERCISES

Carrying things and rotation are huge parts of human movement that often get neglected. Whether you're simply carrying your backpack to class or pitching the ninth inning in the state championship, the principles remain the same. We need to be able to control our bodies across multiple planes of motion, despite outside forces. Therefore, apply the following rotational, anti-rotational, and carrying exercises to your programs.

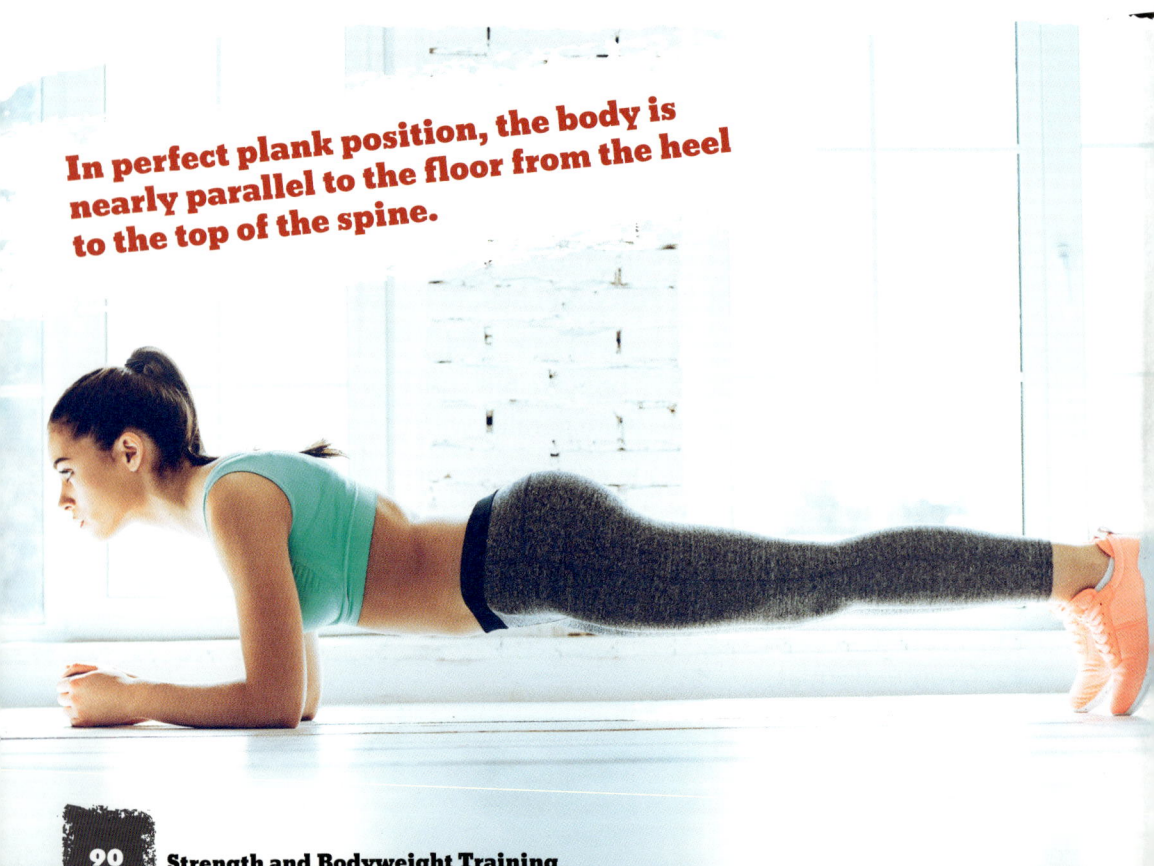

In perfect plank position, the body is nearly parallel to the floor from the heel to the top of the spine.

1. Planks
2. Side planks (with and without rotation)
3. Bird dogs
4. Pallof presses
5. Medicine ball throws
6. Rotational rows
7. Turkish get-ups
8. Farmer's carry
9. Waiter's carry
10. Suitcase carry

For detailed descriptions of each of these exercises, visit the American Council on ACE Exercise Library in the Internet Resources section at the end of this book.

TEXT-DEPENDENT QUESTIONS

1. What is it called when the arm and shoulder blade move together?
2. On which system do quad dominant movements place the most emphasis?
3. Give five examples of rotational or core exercises.

RESEARCH PROJECT

Since weight training has progressed beyond moving one's body weight, multiple lifting implements now exist. Choose one of the three most common—barbell, kettlebell, or dumbbell—and research its history. When was it first invented? By whom? What is it primarily used for? Go into as much detail as you can.

SERIES GLOSSARY OF KEY TERMS

Cardiorespiratory – of or relating to the heart and the respiratory system.

Circuit training – a workout technique involving a series of exercises performed in rotation with minimal rest, often using different pieces of apparatus.

Fatigue – weariness or exhaustion from labor, exertion, or stress.

HDL cholesterol – also known as good cholesterol. A lipoprotein of blood plasma that is composed of a high proportion of protein with little triglyceride and cholesterol and that is correlated with reduced risk of atherosclerosis.

Hormone – a product of living cells that circulates in body fluids (such as blood) and produces a specific and often stimulatory effect on the activity of cells, usually remote from its point of origin.

Lactic acid – a normally present hygroscopic organic acid ($C_3H_6O_3$), especially in muscle tissue, that is a by-product of anaerobic glycolysis, produced in carbohydrate matter usually by bacterial fermentation, and used especially in food and medicine and in industry.

LDL cholesterol – also known as bad cholesterol. A lipoprotein of blood plasma that is composed of a moderate proportion of protein with little triglyceride and a high proportion of cholesterol and that is associated with increased probability of developing atherosclerosis.

Metabolism – the chemical changes in living cells by which energy is provided for vital processes and activities, and new material is assimilated.

Micronutrients – a chemical element or substance (such as calcium or vitamin C) that is essential in minute amounts to the growth and health of a living organism.

Modification – the making of a limited change in something, such as an exercise, that makes the exercise easier.

Physiology – a branch of biology that deals with the functions and activities of life or of living matter (such as organs, tissues, or cells) and of the physical and chemical phenomena involved.

Resistance – of, relating to, or being an exercise involving pushing or pulling against the source of an opposing force (such as a weight) to increase strength.

Tempo – rate of motion or activity.

FURTHER READING

Haff, G. G., and N. T. Triplett. *Essentials of Strength Training and Conditioning.* Champaign: Human Kinetics, 2016.

Kalym, Ashley. *Complete Calisthenics: The Ultimate Guide to Bodyweight Exercise.* 2nd ed. West Sussex, England: Lotus Publishing, 2019.

Rippetoe, Mark. *Starting Strength: Basic Barbell Training.* Wichita Falls: Aasgaard Company, 2017.

Stellabotte, F., and R. Straub. *Weight Training Without Injury: Over 350 Step-By-Step Pictures Including What Not to Do!* Walnut: Regalis Publishing, 2016.

Tumminello, N. *Strength Training for Fat Loss.* Champaign: Human Kinetics, 2014.

INTERNET RESOURCES

American Council on Exercise (ACE)
https://www.acefitness.org/education-and-resources/lifestyle/exercise-library/equipment/no-equipment

ACE is a reputable fitness accreditation organization that provides a library of exercise instruction.

NSCA
www.nsca.com

The National Strength and Conditioning Association, one of the premier governing bodies behind strength training, provides tips on proper strength training technique and programing.

Global Bodyweight Training
https://www.globalbodyweighttraining.com/resources/instructional-articles-and-videos

This website from Global Bodyweight Training offers tutorials and instructional videos on every bodyweight exercise under the sun.

STACK
www.stack.com

STACK is an online, sports performance and athletic resource designed specifically for young athletes.

Stronger By Science
https://www.strongerbyscience.com

Stronger by Science regularly features evidence-based articles by leading experts in the fitness industry about the science of strength training.

INDEX

A
Accessory movements, 50
Actin, 31, 37
"Active for Life" stage, 58–59
"Active Start" stage, 56–57
Agonists, 73
American Academy of Pediatrics, 70
American Orthopaedic Society for Sports Medicine, 70
Ankle injuries
  exercises to preventing, 76
Antagonist, 73
Anterior chain, 88
Arm circles, 23
Athletic performance
  strength training benefits for, 55–56
  See also Long-Term Athlete Development (LTAD) model

B
Backpedaling, 61
Balyi, Istvan, 56, 57
Barbell, 43
Barbell back squat, 89
Barbell bench, 81
Barbell squats, 33
Bench press, 33
Bicep curl, 33
Bicycle crunches, 23
Biomechanics, 21
Body composition
  effects of strength training on, 9
Body strength, building, 24
Bodyweight squats, 88
Bodyweight training, 16, 17, 19–28
  benefits of, 19, 26–28
  closed vs. open kinetic chain movements, 22–23
  functional muscle, building, 20–24
  getting stronger with, 25–26, 48
  goals of strength training, 47–53
    factors manipulation to achieving, 43, 45–46
  resistance training
    to muscle building, 50
    for speed, 50–53
    for strength, 48–50
  strengthening the core, 26–28
  total body strength, building, 24
  training for maximum strength, 48
  and weight training, 43–53
Bone density, 9
Bone fractures, 68–69
Box jumps, 26
"Bracing your core" phrase, 26, 28, 68
Broad jumps, 26

C
Calf raises, 74, 76
Cardiovascular health
  growth and maturation, 12
  neuromuscular development, 10–11

Carrying exercises, 90–91
Centers for Disease Control, 10
Chin-ups, 84
Chu, Donald A., 51, 53
Closed kinetic chain exercises, 22
Cognitive health, 13
Concentric contraction, 33
Coordination, 39–41
Core activation and training, 72–73
Core exercises, 90–91
Core, strengthening, 26–28, 72
Cortisol, 36
CrossFit Games, 85
Crunches, 20
Cutting/lateral running, 61

D
Deadlift, 38, 39
Deceleration/Backpedaling, 61
Density, 46
Depression, 14, 17
Donkey kicks, 23
Dual-energy X-ray absorptiometry (DEXA), 9
Dumbbells, 43

E
Eccentric contraction, 33, 34, 37–38
Elbow/shoulder injuries
  exercises to preventing, 77
Emotional health, 14–17
Endorphins, 13
Epiphyseal plates, 69–70
Exercise
  benefit of, 13
  improving brain function, 13–14
  See also Bodyweight training; Resistance training; Strength training

F
Flutter kicks, 23
Force–velocity curve, 38, 63
Functional muscle, 20–24
  maintaining, 45
"Fundamentals" stage, of LTAD model, 57

G
Glute bridges, 22, 76, 77
Goblet squat, 89
Gorillas, leaning from, 45
Growth hormone, 12, 36
Growth plate issues, 69–70
Growth spurt, 58

H
Hang cleans, 53
Health and wellness benefits, 7
Herniated discs, 68
Hip hinge, 86–87
Hip/lower back injuries
  exercises for preventing, 77

Hopping, 25
Horizontal acceleration, 61
Hypertrophy, 50, 51
  mechanical loading, 35–36
  metabolic stress, 36–37
  muscle damage, 37–38

I
In-season, 65
Injury prevention, 65, 67–77
  ankle, 76
  avoiding injury, 70–71
  bone fractures, 68–69
  core activation and training, 72–73
  elbow/shoulder injuries, 77
  growth plate issues, 69–70
  herniated discs, 68
  hip/low back injuries, 77
  knee, 76
  muscle strain, 67
  regular strength training, 73
  sport-specific prehab, 75–77
  warm-up and mobility, 71–72
Intensity, 46
Inverted row exercise, 22, 82–84
Isometric contraction, 32, 33

J
Journal of Applied Physiology, 13
Journal of Strength and Conditioning Research, 67
Jumping, 25
Junior American Record, 70

K
Kettlebell swings, 43, 53, 87
Knee injuries
  exercises for preventing, 76

L
Lat pulldowns, 36
Lean muscle mass, 9
"Learn to Train" stage, 58
Load vectors, 64
Long-Term Athlete Development (LTAD) model, 56, 59
  stage 1: active start, 56–57
  stage 2: fundamentals, 57
  stage 3: learn to train, 58
  stage 4: train to train, 28
  stage 5: train to compete, 58
  stage 6 and 7: train to win and active for life, 58–59
Lower body hinge, 85–87
  hip hinge/Romanian deadlift, 86–87
  other exercises, 87
Lower body hip dominant, 61
Lower body quad dominant, 61
  barbell back squat, 89
  exercises, 89
Lunges, 24
Lunging, 40, 41

M
Maturation, 12
Max Speed zone, 39
Max Strength zone, 38
Maximum strength, training for, 48
Mechanical loading, 35–36
Mechanosensors, 38
Mental health, 14–17
Metabolic stress, from resistance training, 36–37
Meyer, Gregory, 51, 53
Mitochondria, 35, 36
Mobility, 71–72
Motor units, 31
Movement skills, 57
Muscle, building, 20–24, 34–41, 50
Muscle contraction, 31–33
　concentric, 33
　eccentric, 33
　isometric, 33
Muscle damage, 37–38
Muscle fibers, 31
Muscle strains, 67
Myosin, 31, 38

N
National Strength and Conditioning Association, 7
Neuromuscular control, 10, 11
Neuromuscular system, 39, 40
Neutral spine, 26, 28–29
Nye, Kate, 70

O
Off-season, 64
Open kinetic chain exercises, 22–23

P
Peak height velocity, 58
Peak Power zone, 38
Pelvic positioning, 72
Penn State University, 38
Plank position, 90
Plyometric exercises, 25–26, 27, 50–51, 52, 61
Plyometrics (Chu and Meyer), 51, 53
Post-season, 65
Postural positioning, in weightlifting, 79
Power
　developing, 38–41, 56
　improving with bodyweight training, 25–26, 48
Pre-season, 65
Prehab (pre-rehabilitation), 75–77
Prilepin, Alexander Sergeyevitch, 49
Prilepin's Chart, 49, 62
Progression, 62–63
Proprioception, 22
Proprioceptor, 39
Pull-ups, 20, 22, 24, 47, 48, 84
Pulled muscles. *See* Muscle strains
Push-ups, 20, 22, 79–81

Q
Quad dominant movements, 88–89

R
Regular strength training, 8, 73
Repetitions, 45, 46
Reps, 62–63
Resistance training, 10–11
　to building muscle, 34–41, 50
　coordination and practice, 39–41
　hypertrophy, 35–38
　motor units, 31
　muscle contraction, 31–33
　science behind, 31–41
　for speed, 50–53
　for strength, 48–50
　strength and power training, 38–39
Reverse fly, 23
Romanian deadlifts, 22, 86–87
Rotational exercises, 90–91
Rotational movement, 61
Rowing, 34

S
Scapulohumeral rhythm, 79
Science and Practice of Strength Training (Zatsiorsky), 38
Sets, 45, 46, 62–63
Side-lying leg raises, 23
Single-arm pull-up, 48
Spartans, 35
Specific Adaptation to Imposed Demands (SAID) principle, 35, 70
Speed, 38–41
　resistance training for, 50–53
　weight training for, 53
Speed–Strength zone, 39
Split squats, 22, 24
Sport skills, 58
Sport-specific prehab, 75–77
Sports Medicine journal, 9
Sprinting, 50, 60
Squats, 22, 24, 25, 88
Strength plan
　developing for young athletes, 59–61
Strength training
　barbell bench, 81
　benefits of, 7, 55–56
　bone density, 9
　cardiovascular health, 10–12
　competitive season, 64–65
　developing strength plan, 59–61
　effects on body composition, 9
　exercises, 79–91
　force–velocity curve, 63
　importance of, 7–17
　lean muscle mass, 9
　long-term athlete development, stages of, 56–59
　lower body hinge, 85–87
　lower body quad dominant, 88–89
　optimizing mental and emotional health, 13–17
　other upper body pushing options, 81–82
　and power training, 38–39
　Prilepin's Chart for, 62
　push-up, 79–81
　regular, 73
　resistance training, 48–50
　rotational/carrying/core exercises, 90–91
　sets/reps/progression, 62–63
　upper body pull, 82–85
　upper body push, 79
　for young athletes, 55–65
Strength–Speed zone, 38
Stress strength training, 10

T
Tears, 67
Testosterone, 36
Thoracic positioning, 72
Top-speed sprinting, 61
Total body strength, building, 20, 24
"Train to Compete" stage, 58
"Train to Train" stage, 28
"Train to Win" stage, 58–59
Triceps dip, 49
Trunk injuries, 67
Twisting, 61

U
Upper body pull, 61
　inverted row, 82–84
　other options, 85
　pull-ups/chin-ups, 84
Upper body push, 61, 79
　options, 81–82

V
Vertical jumps, 26, 61
Volume, 46

W
Warm-up, 71–72
Weight training
　vs. bodyweight training, 43–53
Weighted jumps, 53
Well-rounded strength training program, 43, 44
World Health Organization, 14

Y
Young athletes
　benefits from strength training, 55–56
　developing strength plan for, 59–61
Youth strength training, benefits of, 7

Z
Zatsiorsky, Vladimir, 38

AUTHOR BIOGRAPHY

Kimber Rozier is a NSCA certified strength and conditioning specialist who holds dual Bachelor's degrees in Exercise and Sport Science and Spanish, as well as a professional athlete competing with the USA women's national rugby team. In 2013, she earned a bronze medal at the Rugby 7s Women's World Cup in Moscow, and competed in the 2014 15s World Cup in Paris and 2017 World Cup in Ireland. As an entrepreneur, former Harvard coach, and decorated professional rugby player, she loves sharing her knowledge through coaching and writing. Certified by the NSCA and Precision Nutrition, she brings her wealth of experience to the page, sharpening the lens by which we see the world. She writes for multiple small health and wellness businesses, as well as large publications such as Men's Health, MyFitnessPal, and EliteFTS. She now owns her own business, Dare Performance, in which she promotes a healthy lifestyle through journalism.

PHOTO CREDITS

Shutterstock.com: Pg. 1: Jacob Lund, 3: PM production, 6, 23, 85, 88: fizkes, 8: Burnt Red Hen, 18: BublikHaus, 20, 76: Maridav, 21: Jasminko Ibrakovic, 25: Syda Productions, 27: Jon Osumi, 28: Francesco Milanese, 30, 52: WoodysPhotos, 32: vladee, 34: Dean Drobot, 36: need, 37: CI Photos, 39: UfaBizPhoto, 40: Dragon Images, 42: Ivan Kochergin, 44: Prostock-studio, 45: Bojan656, 47: MilanMarkovic78, 49: Philip Date, 51: Serghei Starus, 52: WoodysPhotos, 54: nullplus, 56: JoeSAPhotos, 57: Lucky Business, 59: Monkey Business Images, 60: Surasak_Photo, 62: EduardSV, 63: James A Boardman, 64: JoeSAPhotos, 66: November27, 68: gualtiero boffi, 69: Andrey_Popov, 71: Blanscape, 72: TORWAISTUDIO, 74: Alan Poulson Photography, 75: Mark Nazh, 78, 90: G-Stock Studio, 80: antoniodiaz, 82: nd3000, 83: Jasminko Ibrakovic, 84: michaeljung, 87: Lyashenko Egor

Dreamstime.com: Pg. 10: 7active Studio, 11: Oksun70, 12: Ammentorp, 14: Dave Bredeson, 15: Artofphoto, 16: Maksim Bogdanets

EDUCATIONAL VIDEO LINKS

Chapter 1: http://x-qr.net/1LLQ
Chapter 2: http://x-qr.net/1LaP
Chapter 3: http://x-qr.net/1J3J
Chapter 4: http://x-qr.net/1LBT
Chapter 5: http://x-qr.net/1JBv
Chapter 6: http://x-qr.net/1KpM
Chapter 7: http://x-qr.net/1K33